Praise for *The Planted Runner*

"Plant-based running is more than a diet or a hobby, it's a lifestyle. Claire Bartholic understands this, and in *The Planted Runner* she takes a refreshingly holistic approach to providing the wisdom, encouragement, and inspiration needed to maximize the many benefits of this increasingly popular lifestyle choice."
—*Matt Fitzgerald, award-winning endurance sports journalist and bestselling author of* 80/20 Running *and* How Bad Do You Want It

....

"Whether you are brand new to plant-based eating and running or simply looking to refine how you already fuel and train, Claire Bartholic's *The Planted Runner* has you covered. With joy, passion, and years of experience as a coach, Bartholic offers readers a clear and practical guide."
—*Danielle Friedman, author of* Let's Get Physical: How Women Discovered Exercise and Reshaped the World *and award-winning journalist for the* New York Times

....

"Even if you are not a plant-based runner, Claire Bartholic provides one of the best summaries of running training principles we have ever seen! The book is a smart and fun cheat code for understanding training principles that can help anyone become a better runner or coach. Claire rocks!"
—*David Roche and Megan Roche, MD, authors of* The Happy Runner *and coaches of the Some Work, All Play team*

....

"I suspect many runners have toyed with the idea of switching to a plant-based diet but have hesitated or reverted because of concerns that this change would negatively affect their running performance. Claire has written an excellent book that provides both sound training wisdom along with plant-based nutritional guidance showing that there is no inconsistency between running at one's best while following a plant-based diet. I would have loved to have had this resource when I started my plant-based journey 13 years ago!"
—*Dan King, M60 American, world-record holder in the mile, and plant-based athlete*

....

"Claire Batholic's humor, insights, and gentle demeanor make her the ideal guide for those navigating all the highs and lows that every new runner encounters."
—*Josiah Hesse, bestselling author of* Runner's High *and journalist for* Vice, Esquire, *and* The Guardian

....

"This is a really comprehensive text that gives the beginner (and not-so-beginner!) runner great practical advice about how to get the most out of the time they are running. From mindset, nutrition, and training advice, this book really highlights Claire's knowledge about running. Do yourself a favor, and pick up a copy."
–*Dr. Eoin Everard, PhD, five-time Irish National Champion and current 3k Masters European Champion*

....

"Ever since I started running, I've been all over the place with how I fuel my body, so I was very much in need of a book like *The Planted Runner*. It's straightforward, filled with expert advice, and, most important to me, it's written from a place of no judgment! This book is a helpful resource that I can pick and choose from, knowing that anything I incorporate will be helpful to my health and my training."
–*Erin Azar, humorist, running advocate, and social media superstar*

....

"In her debut book, Boston Marathon qualifier, state Master's Marathon Champion, competitive master's athlete, and certified running coach Claire Bartholic offers a comprehensive yet accessible running guide. But don't let the title fool you. *The Planted Runner* covers much more than nutrition. In addition to recipes, Bartholic includes training tips and mindset reframes for a volume packed with helpful, science-based information. While the book is intended for plant-based athletes, it offers splendid advice for anyone hoping to run their best race at any age. Read this book and meet your goals while enjoying both the sport and the food."
–*Nita Sweeney, award-winning author of* Make Every Move a Meditation

....

"A fantastic read for any runner interested in a healthy, plant-based life! A comprehensive beginner's guide with practical tips to not only eat and recover, but also to train, race, and prepare for any running challenge."
–*Brodie Sharpe, BhlthSci, MPhysioPrac, APAM, physiotherapist, host of the Run Smarter podcast*

....

Claire Bartholic

The Planted RUNNER

Running Your Best With Plant-Based Nutrition

Meyer & Meyer Sport

British Library of Cataloguing in Publication Data
A catalogue record for this book is available from the British Library

The Planted Runner
Maidenhead: Meyer & Meyer Sport (UK) Ltd., 2023
ISBN: 978-1-78255-246-8

© 2023 by Meyer & Meyer Sport (UK) Ltd.
Aachen, Auckland, Beirut, Cairo, Cape Town, Dubai, Hägendorf, Hong Kong, Indianapolis, Maidenhead, Manila, New Delhi, Singapore, Sydney, Tehran, Vienna
Member of the World Sport Publishers' Association (WSPA), www.w-s-p-a.org
Printed by Print Consult GmbH, Munich, Germany
Printed in Slovakia

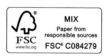

ISBN: 978-1-78255-246-8
Email: info@m-m-sports.com
www.thesportspublisher.com

Contents

Introduction

How I went from wanting to look good at my high school reunion to becoming a 2:58 marathoner and running coach

I just wanted to look good at my high school reunion. Little did I know my vanity would change my entire life.

I was one of those forgettable types in high school: not pretty enough to be popular, too smart to be cool, not nerdy enough to be brainy. I floated in between the cliques fairly easily, always blending, yet never belonging.

When the 20th year reunion plans started coming together on Facebook, I immediately felt the need to go back to my hometown and be everything I wasn't in high school. I imagined gliding through the rented event space past clusters of foil balloons decorated with "Class of 1993," Duran Duran playing softly in the background, looking beautiful, successful, and confident.

I had the successful part down. At the time, I was married with two healthy kids, we lived in a lovely home, and I had a thriving real estate career. But for some deep reason that I can't quite explain, I wanted nothing more than to make a knock-your-socks off impression in front of my old classmates.

Now, I wasn't what anyone but a Hollywood producer would call fat. A few months earlier, I had started following a whole foods, plant-based diet and that was beginning to help me lose some extra weight. But mostly, I had your average, mom-of-two-young-kids-with-a-stressful-career body: soft, stretched out, and a little rounder and puffier than it used to be. Not bad, but not knock-your-socks-off.

So, I started running.

Running Is an Acquired Taste and I Didn't Like It (At First)

I had dabbled a little in running a couple times in my life, but it had never really stuck. I ran a half marathon one fall in my 20s in an attempt to get over a painful breakup. But I couched my running habit with the onset of cold weather and the reconciliation with my ex, who later became my husband (who later became my ex).

I knew running would be the quickest means to the end I wanted (to look hot for people I used to know a million years ago).

But I hated nearly every step.

When I'd leave the house to go on a run, my husband would call out supportively, "have fun!" More often than not, I'd snarl back, "Fun? I'm going running. I'm not having fun. Running sucks."

And running did suck. Every single time. But it worked. Along with carefully eliminating everything that tasted good from my diet, I lost a handful of pounds in time for the reunion. I got the compliments from the popular kids and the smart kids that my 16-year-old self so desperately wanted 20 years earlier.

Honestly, I looked great. I had achieved my primary goal and could stop the torture. But for some reason, I kept running. I was feeling strong in my new body and thought maybe I should try running that half marathon again, just to see how it would go. So I did. And I beat the time I had gotten ten years earlier by about seven minutes, which felt amazing.

As I shared my accomplishment on social media, I began to pay attention to other runners in my network. One acquaintance from high school (who didn't go to the reunion) mentioned that she was training for the Boston Marathon.

And so, right then and there, my sights were set on running Boston.

The Road to the Marathon

I quickly learned that you can't just run Boston because you want to; you have to qualify by running another marathon first in a certain time graded for your age. I needed to run a marathon fast, so I picked the one in my backyard in the mountains of North Carolina held the following spring.

Now, most experienced runners would say that there is nothing about running a marathon in the mountains that is going to be fast. And certainly not one held in March when it could be 15 degrees and snowing, or worse, 40 degrees and pouring rain.

But I was not an experienced runner and signed up anyway, boldly planning to qualify for Boston on my very first try.

Yeah, that didn't happen.

Once I was signed up, I was all in. Enthusiastically, I dove down the online rabbit hole of information on how to train for and run a marathon. I learned about weekly mileage, long run progression, and interval training. I found a free training plan from a company called RunnersConnect that told me exactly what I needed to do to run a 3:30 marathon, which was 10 minutes faster than what I needed to qualify for Boston.

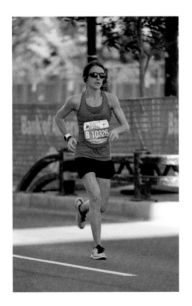

I did it all. But it didn't work.

Race day was cold and rainy and I fell apart somewhere around mile 18 and had to walk/jog to the finish. I crossed the line in a respectable 4:02, which was 22 minutes short of what I needed.

Missing my mark by so much lit a fire in me. I don't know where my belief came from, but I knew that I could have finished in time, if I had only done a few things differently. I just knew that I could be much, much faster.

I was hooked.

One day, I saw an ad for a race outside of Salt Lake City, Utah. This was also a mountain race, but in only one direction: downhill. Surely, I could qualify there. I signed up and followed my free plan again. This time, however, it worked.

My legs had gotten a little stronger, my speed a little faster, and my long runs were a little easier. I started eating all the plant foods that would nourish and support my running instead of restricting calories for weight loss.

Running was no longer something I was doing to change my appearance but instead something that gave me strength and purpose. I wasn't running; I was training.

I crossed the finish line in Utah with just 90 seconds to spare. I used every ounce of that strength I had built to earn my goal time. And I was ecstatic to be able to race the Boston Marathon the following April, tears of joy mixing with the cold rain on my face as I lopped yet another 12 minutes off my personal best.

Beyond Boston

Fueled by the exhilarating sense of accomplishment from my hard work, I continued to train and race two marathons a year for the next four years. Each race I progressively lowered my time and earned a Masters Champion title along the way.

My final marathon came in 64 minutes faster than my first. I went from a finish time of 4:02 all the way to 2:58:41 at age 42.

I am often asked how I was able to progress so quickly, from someone who didn't run to a champion Masters athlete that could run 26.2 miles in less than three hours.

Is it genetics? Special training? Hidden talent?

Sure, there has to be at least a little genetic ability in me, but maybe not as much as you'd think. My dad was a life-long recreational runner, diligently marking his three morning miles on a wall calendar in the kitchen every other day.

But there are no elite athletes in my family tree. Far from it in fact.

The reason that I was so successful in running marathons came down to equal parts passion and desire for accomplishment. Running still sucked at times, but I loved

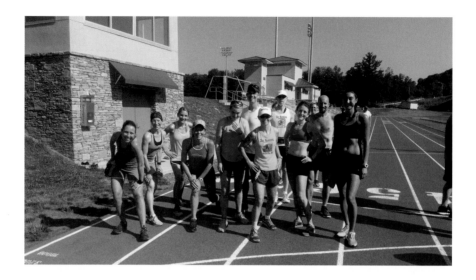

that the more I worked at running, the better I got. I loved learning everything that I could about how to run and train better and eventually hired the coaches at RunnersConnect to help me take my training even further.

Soon I joined running groups in town and found a tribe of like-minded people who were as obsessed with running as I was. I added strength training twice a week and trail running once a week. Gradually, I started building my weekly mileage up from 30 to 40 to 60 miles per week, eventually regularly clocking months of 70- and 80-mile weeks. Finally, I topped out at 90 miles in a single week.

In a typical week, I ran a hard track session on Tuesday with the running group, a fast-tempo run ending at a brewery on Thursday, a medium-length, medium-fast run on Saturday, and a long run of up to 22 miles on Sunday. The days in between were slower, coming in at 8 to10 miles.

I rarely took a day off and rarely got injured.

Yes, it was a lot.

From Athlete to Coach

While still competing in marathons, I became a coach myself at RunnersConnect. They truly are an expert team and taught me so much valuable information that I still use today.

Eventually, I decided to branch out on my own with my coaching business, The Planted Runner. I've learned that it's not just running that will help you become the best athlete you can be. You also need to fuel your body optimally and train your mindset, all of which I emphasize with my athletes.

Not everyone I coach is as "all-in" as I was as a runner, but we all share the love of running and how it can transform our lives.

As an athlete, I don't train as hard as I used to. I find far more joy from helping others achieve their dreams than I ever did for myself. My passion is no longer to see how fast or how far I can run myself, but to help other runners become their very best.

I still love to run and may race again someday. But it will be for pure joy and not the numbers on the clock. Don't get me wrong, being a fit and strong runner is something I never want to get away from, but my running has greater purpose now.

Not to mention, I'll still want to look good at my next reunion.

How a Whole Foods Plant-Based Diet Factored In to My Success

I went plant-based before I was a serious runner.

One night in November 2012, I sat down to watch the documentary *Forks Over Knives*. To say it changed my life is an understatement. From that day forward, I knew that living a whole foods, plant-based life made the most sense for my health first and the planet second.

While that movie was eye-opening for me, I don't take its findings as the only "right" way to live for everyone. The research that I've read since seems to indicate that if you decide to only be 80 to 90 percent whole foods plant-based (WFPB), your health will dramatically improve over the standard American diet.

But I'm not an 80 to 90 percent kind of person; I'm either 100 percent or nothing. I like to have clear guidelines when it comes to my life as much as possible and simply avoiding anything that came from an animal works best for me.

Now that doesn't mean I don't indulge in vegan junk food like potato chips or sweets on occasion (life is too short for that!). But when I do, I also try to balance it with lots of whole plant foods as well.

When it comes to fueling your body best for athletic training, there's lots of evidence that whole plants do an amazing job, and I'll get into that soon. Is it a coincidence that I was able to train so hard for years in my late 30s/early 40s and never get injured? Was it the plants? There's no scientific way to know for sure, but they definitely helped!

Guiding Your Success

Now that you've learned a little about me, the rest of this book is for you. I developed this book from years of coaching athletes, interviewing experts, and researching the science behind endurance running, mindset training, and fueling with plants. My goal is for this to be a way to help anyone who would like to learn to run better, fuel better, and feel better.

You'll learn about why a whole plant diet can be so beneficial for your health and so effective for athletes (and everyone else!). You don't have to be 100 percent vegan or plant-based to improve your health, but thriving on a delicious, whole-foods diet might just be easier than you think!

Then we'll explore how to begin a running habit no matter where you are in your fitness journey. I don't think there is a single runner on the planet that loves every single run they have ever run. Running will always have an element of challenge to it, no matter how good you get, but there are many ways to make running easier and more fun.

Fueling your runs properly is essential to both feeling and performing your best. You'll learn how to fuel your runs with the best foods for health and performance (and you'll learn when not to!). We'll go over hydration tips, the best recovery foods, and how to use running and nutrition to lose fat and gain muscle.

Once you have the essentials down, we will move on to basic training techniques and building on your skills. You'll learn how to add mileage, work on your speed, and tap into the specific training that you'll need to get better at any distance.

But you can't be your best on running alone. Strength, balance, and mobility training are all important elements for any well-rounded runner. I'll go over exactly what you need (good news: it's not that much!) and how it helps.

Now, all of this great training and nutrition will only get you so far if you don't take the time to recover. Solid recovery after workout is how the body repairs and builds from the damage done by working your muscles hard.

Next comes mindset training. It's clear that to be your best at anything that's difficult, you have to get your mind on board. I'll go over the exact mindset techniques that I use with my personal athletes that help banish negative self-talk and bolster self-confidence.

And finally, let's get you ready to race! For many runners, racing well can be an immensely satisfying experience that caps off a successful training cycle. But a great race doesn't happen by accident. Racing is a skill that you will need to practice, and I'll explore the proven strategies that will lead to your fastest race time.

Even if racing is not your ultimate goal with your running, training your body and mind like an athlete can have benefits that go beyond a single race. Your body will become stronger and faster, and you will gain the confidence that only comes from learning to do something hard well!

Chapter One

Improve Endurance, Heart Health, and Recovery With Plants

 How switching to a whole plant diet can help you control your weight and feel better in your body

Often I say "everyone's vegan when they are running." You don't see too many people fueling their marathons with milkshakes and cheeseburgers (well, maybe ultrarunners do!), so it's normal to wonder if you should be fueling without meat and dairy all the time.

It's never been easier (or trendier!) to move to a plant-based diet. No longer an obscure way of life for determined hippies, more and more people are choosing to eat more plants more often. Plant-based foods fill the grocery store shelves, dominate the dairy section, and even show up on menus at most restaurants.

But is this different way of eating actually healthy? Can you really fuel your life and your running with plants only?

The evidence (and the anecdotes) overwhelmingly say yes. Plant-based runners like Scott Jurek, Michael Wardian, Ellie Greenwood, Fiona Oakes, Rich Roll, Brendan Brazier, and yours truly have consistently topped podiums and broken records, running entirely on plants.

But will it work for you?

In this section, I'm going to cover

- the benefits that a plant-based diet provides runners;
- the potential downsides to going plant-based; and
- a day in the life of a vegan runner with meal examples that you can try today.

The terms in this discussion can be a little confusing or misleading, so let me first go over some definitions.

Vegan is the simplest to define. It means that you do not eat anything that comes from an animal. For many vegans, their first priority is animal rights, so they do not buy wool, leather, or even drink wine that has been traditionally processed using animal products. This also leaves a lot of clearly unhealthy vegan foods on the table like cookies, sugary sodas, and greasy potato chips, because, again, health is not the main reason for being a vegan. It's not about what you eat as a vegan, but rather about what you do not eat.

Vegetarians skip the meat but might include eggs or dairy products. *Plant-based* means that your diet is based in plants, preferably as unprocessed as possible, but you might not be 100% vegan. You might have some fish for dinner or maybe an egg every once in a while, but the vast majority of your food is plant-based.

There's not really an agreed-on term for a 100% plant-based eater. Some people just say vegan because it's easier to understand, others say "strictly plant-based," which doesn't sound very nice to me. So for the purposes of this book, I use the term *plant-based* to mean someone who's eating mostly or entirely plants. And, actually, the science tells us that even if we are not 100% plant-based, it's more about what you do eat, not really about what you don't.

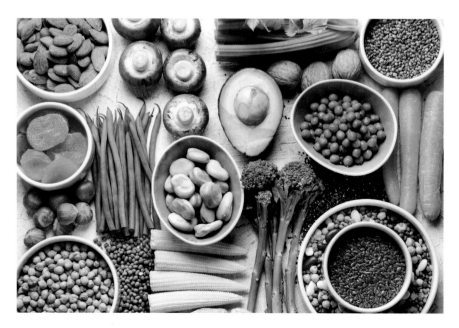

I've been entirely plant-based for 10 years. I choose to eat this way because I am convinced of the health benefits, and it works for me. I have educated myself on what it takes to build a healthy plant-based diet, and I've learned the common pitfalls that can make a well-meaning plant-curious eater go running back to their meat and cheese.

The main reason for me is my health and well-being, but it's also pretty cool that this way of eating is far gentler on the planet and, of course, the animals.

I am also a certified sports nutrition specialist, which means that I am qualified to coach nutrition for athletes, but I do want to make it 100% clear that I am not a registered dietitian. If you are really struggling with your nutrition and need detailed meal plans, you should search out an RD that works with runners.

Disclaimers out of the way, I've compiled here the science that can help you decide whether a fully or even partially plant-based diet is right for you and your running.

A 2019 study[1] in the medical journal *Nutrients* looked at plant-based endurance athletes and their overall health. The researchers wanted to know if these athletes could truly thrive and perform only on plants. They determined that it was not only possible, but that a plant-based diet had some unique advantages, which I cover in the following section.

Benefits of a Plant-Based Diet
Reduced Inflammation

The first amazing effect of a plant-based diet is reduced inflammation.

When you come back from a tough run or strength-training session, your body's immediate response is inflammation. This is actually a good thing. Acute inflammation is your body's way of calling in the troops to assess and repair the damage you've done. We want this process to happen, but we also want it to be over pretty quickly. If you are still inflamed when you are ready for your next workout, you will likely be sore, tired, and your performance will suffer.

A plant-based diet could be an important way to help reduce inflammation. Taking a look at 18 prior studies in a 2017 meta-analysis[2], vegetarian diets consumed over a two-year period were shown to reduce certain markers of inflammation. This suggests that there is an anti-inflammatory effect of plant-based foods.

The researchers theorized that the anti-inflammatory benefits of plant-based diets may have stemmed from their antioxidant content, the absence of things that may be inflammatory, or the absence of pro-inflammatory fats.

A few studies have examined the possibility that specific foods with antioxidant activity might decrease the inflammation response and promote recovery like tart cherries[3], pomegranates[4], blueberries[5], blackcurrants[6], and watermelon[7]. Another good reason to load up on fruit after your workout!

Improved Cardiovascular Health

The next area in which more plants can be advantageous is your cardiovascular health. As a runner, your heart is working hard every day to pump blood to your muscles. You know that your heart is probably already healthier than your non-running peers. But did you know that well-trained endurance runners are actually at a higher risk for certain heart conditions? And the risk increases as we age.

In a surprising study done in the UK in 2017[8], coronary plaques were found in 44% of middle-aged and older endurance athletes engaged in cycling or running, compared to 22% of sedentary controls. And in a study[9] of 50 men who had run at least 25 consecutive Twin Cities Marathons, the runners were found to have increased total plaque volume, calcified plaque volume, and non-calcified plaque volume compared to 23 sedentary controls. It seems that the more marathons you run, the greater the degree of myocardial damage.

Now, before you stop running to save your heart, the important thing to remember is that sudden cardiac death while running is very rare. But why are these older athletes experiencing cardiac damage? Is it from the running or from the foods they use to fuel it?

The answers are not entirely clear, but what has been shown is that increased consumption of animal products with higher levels of saturated fats, cholesterol, and relative absence of antioxidants and fiber may contribute to atherosclerotic changes. So if you are replacing the calories that you burn running with lots of heart-unhealthy foods, your heart might not be able to take it. Not to mention, if your arteries are restricted with plaque, that restricts blood flow to both your brain and your muscles, ultimately hurting your running performance.

Better Glycogen Storage

The next cool part of a plant-based diet for runners is better glycogen storage. Glycogen is the fuel that our bodies make from the food we eat and that fuels our brains and our muscles. We store glycogen mainly in the muscles and liver, and the more you have on board, the farther and faster you can run without hitting the dreaded wall.

But the surprising fact is that most endurance athletes aren't filling up their glycogen tanks enough. Sure, if you are an experienced marathon runner, you've probably learned to carbo load in the days before a race, but what I'm talking about is chronic carbohydrate underfueling[10]. This eating pattern will put you at risk for an overly rapid depletion of glycogen from the muscles and liver, making you feel fatigued on your runs much sooner than you would when fully fueled.

A 2016 study[11] of athletes participating in full and half Ironman triathlons, winter triathlons, and winter pentathlons showed that only 46% reported meeting the recommended carbohydrate intake for athletes training one to three hours per day. That's about ≥6 grams of carbs/kg body weight per day. Grains, fruit, legumes, and root vegetables are rich in complex carbohydrates, so athletes who go plant-based can typically hit those marks much more easily.

Better Blood Flow and Increased Tissue Oxygenation

Runners can also expect better blood flow and increased oxygenation of tissues on a plant-based diet. As a runner, your blood is likely already a little thinner with a little more plasma than a sedentary couch potato. Blood this has low viscosity can move through your body easier and oxygenate your tissues better, which leads to better running performance. Your food choices also play an important role in the viscosity of your blood as well. And guess what helps the most? Yep, plants.

In a study[12] comparing 48 individuals following vegetarian eating patterns and 41 matched controls, plasma viscosity, cell volume, and blood viscosity were lower in vegetarians, and the stricter the avoidance of animal products, the greater the observed differences. The entirely plant-based subjects had significantly lower blood viscosity compared to those having meat less than once a week.

So is it the plants that are providing the benefit to your blood and arteries? Or is the culprit the fat from the animal products? What about plant fats and oils? Studies[13] have shown animal fat to impair the flexibility of your arteries, but the results are mixed as they pertain to olive oil[14,15,16]. So to stay in the clear, it's likely best to get your fats from whole plants like nuts, seeds, and avocados.

Leaner Body Mass

Finally, the benefit that many people get most excited about is that a plant-based diet can help keep you lean.

Researchers have concluded that it's easier to have a lean body mass when you are only eating whole plant foods versus a traditional omnivore diet[20]. Fruits, veggies, beans, and whole grains all are much denser in nutrients per calorie than meat and most dairy products. They are also full of water and fiber, so you can fill up and be satisfied with far fewer calories per bite.

A typical plant-based diet is much lower in fat than a standard diet and that can have a dramatic effect on your metabolism. In a 2005 study[17], the use of a low-fat vegan diet for 14 weeks increased the energy burn after eating by 16%. The scientists theorized that this was due to changes at the mitochondrial and cellular levels.

To oversimplify a complex process, the mitochondria and the gut bacteria end up increasing energy expenditure. And there is a greater metabolic cost of converting dietary carbohydrate to body fat when compared to converting dietary fat to body fat[18]. In other words, carbohydrates from plants are easier to burn as fuel and harder to store as fat, leading to a leaner body without trying too hard.

A leaner body is easier to move around, can boost your VO2 max[19], and will often make you a faster runner—up to a point of course. If you are already at a healthy weight, your training will make a far bigger difference than changes in your body weight. But if you can lose extra fat by simply choosing healthier foods that satisfy you, that is certainly a good thing.

Be Sure to Make it Delicious!

Your tastebuds will likely start to change as you eat more and more plants. Processed foods are intentionally hyper-delicious to keep you coming back for more. As you eliminate those, you'll soon start to notice the incredible taste of a perfectly ripe pineapple or a deliciously flavored veggie stir fry.

And speaking of delicious, don't forget to make it delicious! When I first went plant-based, I was so focused on making everything so healthy that everything tasted terrible! You can make simple, rich flavors with sauces and seasonings that even a carnivore will love.

Downsides of a Plant-Based Diet

At this point, you might be thinking that if all the evidence is so strong for a plant-based diet, why aren't more elite athletes plant-based? There are a lot of reasons for this, both social and practical. It can be inconvenient to be 100% plant-based. And the honest truth is that a plant-based diet isn't a magic bullet. Lots and lots of athletes reach the very top of their sports while choosing to include meat and dairy. But what the science says is that at the very least, a well-planned plant-based diet can be just as effective as a well-planned omnivorous diet for athletic performance[21]. Even with all the great reasons why plants can help your running, it's still important to understand the downsides and pitfalls.

Social

The first drawback is purely social. If everyone around you eats differently than you, it can be hard to be the odd one out. But, if you are reading this book, you are likely someone who's interested in something a little bit different: long-distance running. You are probably already used to going against the grain a little bit, so if you can do that, you certainly can shift to eating more plants!

Where to Start

The next pitfall is not really knowing where to start. If you simply remove the chicken from your plate and replace it with bread or lettuce, you're probably going to be disappointed in the whole plant-based thing pretty quickly. You will still want to follow balanced macro practices no matter what diet you choose, meaning you are getting in your requirements for carbs, fat, and protein.

The Protein Question

Once you decide to go plant-based, the most common question you'll get will be, "Where do you get your protein?" The answer is that you can get plenty of protein on a plant-based diet! But you do have to educate yourself on what you are doing. All plant foods contain protein, but athletes require more than non-athletes, so you will have to make conscious protein choices every meal.

My favorites are beans, tofu, lentils, tempeh, quinoa, nuts, and seeds. If you are really struggling to get in enough as a runner, there are some great plant-based protein shakes and bars that can help you hit your marks. Whole foods are best, of course, but progress is far better than perfection.

A very common comment I get when I talk about plant-based protein is that plant proteins are less bioavailable than animal proteins. Or that you can't get all the essential amino acids from each type of protein. Both of those statements are completely true. But those hurdles are also easily overcome by eating a wide variety of plant-based proteins throughout the day to make sure you get enough.

There are a ton of plant-based meat substitutes out there that are delicious and can make your transition easier, but nutritionally, most of the fake meats aren't much healthier than the originals, so save those for an occasional treat rather than using them as staples.

Supplements

A critical piece of information for any plant-based or vegan diet is that you do need to supplement with B12. You might also want to get a blood test to check your levels of iron and vitamin D. B12 is something that many, many people are lacking, not just vegans, and it's a bacteria found in soil that concentrates in animal flesh. With cleaner produce and less fertile soils, it's something most of us can't get enough of without a supplement.

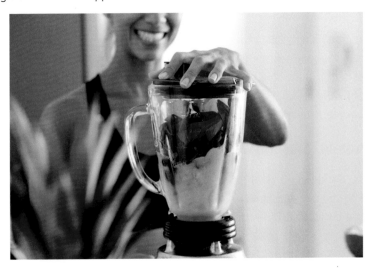

A Day of Eating for a Plant-Based Runner

Now that you know the benefits and what to watch out for, let's look at what a real plant-based diet looks like for a runner. Obviously, it can and will vary depending on your calorie and nutrient needs, but here's a quick example:

Breakfast: Oatmeal made with a fortified plant-based milk, such as almond. Top it with berries, pecans, and a sprinkle of sunflower seeds.

Post-workout snack: Smoothie made with plant-based milk, peanut butter or protein powder, banana, greens, and a dash of chia or hemp seeds.

Lunch: I usually make extra dinner from the night before to make prep super simple and throw everything on a bed of greens. A good example is a loaded salad with greens, red onions, corn, black beans, avocado, salsa, roasted sweet potato with a drizzle of tahini and lime dressing.

Afternoon snack: Fresh fruit with a handful of mixed nuts.

Dinner: Stir fry with brown rice or quinoa, tons of your favorite veggies, crispy tofu, and a swirl of sweet-and-spicy teriyaki sauce.

See? It's not too complicated or weird, is it? There really are a million ways to mix it up and enjoy delicious plant-based foods that are good for you, the planet, and your running.

Six Steps to Become a Whole Foods Plant-Based Runner

Trying a whole food plant-based diet is surely going to be a resolution for a lot of runners this year. Here are six steps to becoming a whole foods plant-based runner that will make the process go a little more smoothly.

1. Examine Your "Why" and Write It Down

There are many reasons for choosing a plant-based or vegan lifestyle, and tapping into why you want to make this choice is essential to sticking with it long term. I'm not going to try to convince you that this is the right choice for you or say you need to be 100 percent vegan, but if you are curious about it, there are lots of ways to learn more.

I committed to plants after watching *Forks Over Knives* in 2012. My main reason is to fuel my body with good food that will enable me to live a long and active life. Then I learned more about the intense environmental impact animal agriculture causes to our land, air, and seas. Knowing I was not a part of the system made it even easier to stick to my personal health goals.

For me, animal welfare is not my primary motivation, but for some vegans, it is, and it can be incredibly powerful. No one really wants to talk about the atrocities that we commit on other sentient beings, and I won't get into it here, but if this is your "why," it is certainly a good one.

2. Decide If You Are an All-Or-Nothing or Incremental Changer

Personally, I thrive on rules and routine. The fewer decisions I have to make, the easier things are. So I'm an All-or-Nothing. When I went fully plant-based, that was that (okay, I do admit to stealing some of my kids' Goldfish right at the beginning, but that was short-lived). To be fair, I was pretty close to being vegetarian already, so it wasn't like I went from hamburgers to tofu in one day, but once I made the commitment, there was no turning back.

Other people do not find the transition so simple and need to ease into it. I recommend that you start eliminating the animal foods that you don't especially like in the first place. For many people, that's cows and pigs. Once that feels comfortable, you can excuse the birds and fish and see how that goes.

The hardest to give up is usually eggs and dairy since they are so prevalent in our food supply and because...cheese. We are wired to love something that is fatty, salty, and umami, and cheese hits all those cravings. But if you are armed with healthier alternatives made from plants, you might find that it ends up being easier than you think to go all in on a whole foods plant-based lifestyle as a runner.

3. Arm Yourself With Really Tasty Plant-Based Swaps

Even if your "why" is because a whole foods plant-based diet is one of the healthiest in the world, don't forget to make it taste good! My biggest mistake starting out was to make sure everything I made was so ridiculously healthy that taste was secondary. My family began to hate my cooking and resent this change that I was "forcing" on them. So I finally got some good cookbooks that focused on flavor, which made my cooking something even an omnivore could love.

4. Focus on Simple, Whole Foods

It's never been easier to go vegan than it is today. Grocery stores stock an amazing array of meat alternatives that are surprisingly good, but many are not really nutritional superstars. Better to think of those as occasional treats rather than staples. Runners can often be the type to overcomplicate things, so do your best to keep it simple. Fruit and nuts make a quick, nutritious snack that is the perfect recovery food right after a run. I love a medjool date filled with a smear of almond butter! For dinner, it doesn't get a whole lot easier (or inexpensive) than beans and rice with greens. Spice it up with taco seasoning for a Mexican flair, or try a spicy peanut sauce with flavors of Southeast Asia. There are a world of possibilities!

5. Think About Protein, But Don't Obsess About It

All plant food contains protein, so as long as you are taking in enough calories, you are likely getting enough protein. But different types of plants contain different amino acids, so you do want to make sure you are eating a variety of foods.

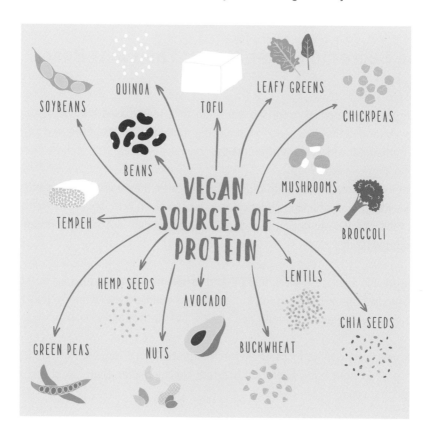

Athletes, however, have a higher protein need than sedentary people. The Academy of Nutrition and Dietetics, Dietitians of Canada, and the American College of Sports Medicine recommend 1.2 to 2.0 grams of protein per kilogram of body weight per day for athletes, depending on training. I discuss this more in the section on protein in this chapter.

6. Supplement With B12

One thing that is difficult to obtain naturally in a vegan diet is B12, so supplementing is a very good idea. B12 is produced by bacteria found in soil, and it's more concentrated in animal flesh than in plants.

With modern farming, our soil has been depleted of this natural resource, so even non-vegans are likely to be deficient.

Moving to a whole plant diet can be life-changing for you, the planet, and clearly, the animals. It doesn't have to be complicated, and you don't have to be perfect to see a difference in how you feel and, eventually, how you look and perform.

The Secret to Better Meals: The Plant-Based Plate

Once you've decided to make the transition to a plant-based lifestyle, it can be really exciting at first. You head to the grocery store pumped about this new journey into optimum health and then you realize...you have no idea what you are doing.

I've found that many people struggle initially because they simply cut out meat and dairy without really thinking about what to replace them with. Bread and pasta are easy fallbacks and can quickly lead to an unbalanced diet (not to mention they get old pretty quickly).

Some people find themselves hungry and unsatisfied because in their quest for supreme health, they eat nothing but salad for a couple days. Naturally, they then become super hungry and cranky and quickly lose motivation.

It becomes very easy to focus on all the things you "can't" eat, get frustrated, and then end up right back where you started, declaring that plant-based just isn't working for you.

There is a better way!

The key to a successful, healthy, and delicious plant-based diet is knowing how to make your meals satisfying, well-balanced, and delicious. And it just might be easier than you think.

I like to build my plant-based meals while thinking about a dinner plate. Half the plate gets filled with vegetables and/or fruits, 25 percent is plant-based protein like beans, and 25 percent is whole grains or starchy vegetables like sweet potatoes. Then I add a drizzle of a plant-based fat like tahini or a sprinkle of nuts, and that's it!

Armed with this formula, you can create limitless options for the perfect plant-based meal.

Let's look at our plate in a little more detail.

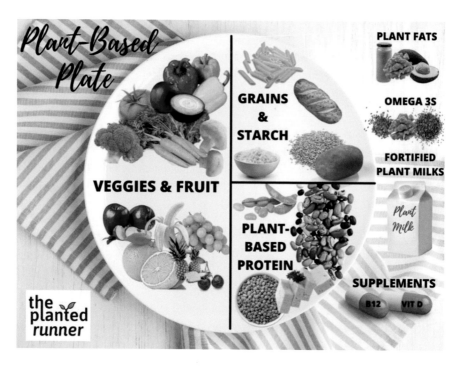

Fruits and Vegetables (50 Percent)

Fruits and vegetables are full of vitamins, minerals, fiber, and antioxidants that can help reduce the risk of developing chronic disease. They also are rich in fiber, which makes you feel fuller longer with fewer calories per bite. Fiber is essential for gut health and digestion.

While some fruits and some vegetables may rank "higher" if you were to put them on a list, the truth is all fruits and vegetables are good for you! You can choose fresh, frozen, or even the convenience of canned. Variety is important, so aim to include a rainbow of different colors as often as you can such as green vegetables (like leafy greens, bok choy, and broccoli) and orange vegetables (like carrots, butternut squash, and bell peppers).

Many guidelines recommend between five to seven servings of fruits and vegetables daily. A serving is the equivalent of about half a cup of fruit or cooked vegetables, which you can have at meals or as snacks.

Starches and Whole Grains (25 Percent)

Starches and whole grains are an important source of long-lasting energy that can also be rich in gut-happy fiber.

Great choices include oatmeal, rice, whole grain breads, wheat/corn tortillas, whole grain pastas, quinoa (technically a seed!), barley, millet, teff, amaranth, buckwheat, sweet potatoes, white potatoes, and corn.

Most dieticians say to aim for at least half of your daily grain servings to be whole grains, but the truth is there is little benefit to highly refined grains. Aim for the majority of your grains to be whole, but allow for some leeway on occasion!

Plant-Based Protein (25 Percent)

Protein is essential for muscle maintenance and growth. The great part about plant-based proteins is that they often are lower in fat and include fiber as well, keeping you fuller longer.

Examples are soy products such as tofu, tempeh, and edamame, seitan, green peas, all beans, chickpeas, and lentils. Other sources that are both protein and fat sources are anything in the nut and seed categories, such as hemp seeds, sunflower seeds, pumpkin seeds, walnuts, almonds, peanuts, and all forms of nut and seed butters. Vegan meat replacements are usually high in protein as well but are typically not whole foods, so enjoy them in moderation.

Make the transition to plant-based simple by straight-up swapping out the protein. Trade dairy milk for soy milk for similar protein profiles, swap out eggs for a tofu scramble, use lentils with taco spices in southwestern dishes, and cook up a big batch of chickpea noodle soup.

Plant-Based Fats

Fat is an essential part of the human diet. It's also one that is very calorie-rich per gram (nine calories per gram versus four for protein and carbohydrate), so a little goes a long way.

All plants contain some amount of fat, and rich, whole food sources include coconut, avocados, and nuts and seeds. Using a small amount of these foods as more of a condiment (rather than a significant portion of your plate) is a great way to keep your meal balanced.

Notice that I didn't include oils in this equation. While some oils (like olive) are considered to be heart healthy, oil is just about as far away from a whole food as you can get. You don't have to avoid oil entirely to stick mainly to a whole foods plant-based diet, but it's something that can get out of hand very quickly, especially if you are trying to lower the fat in your diet. It's far better to get your good fats from real, whole food!

Omega-3s

Speaking of fat, omega-3 fatty acids are an important part of the diet and essential to your health. Most commonly found in fish, you can still achieve your omega-3 goals with plants.

Walnuts, hemp seeds, chia seeds, flax seeds, and even brussels sprouts are good sources. If you don't eat these foods, you may want to consider a plant-based supplement.

Fortified Foods

While it can be fun to make your own oat, almond, or rice milk, fortified plant milks provide many of the vitamins and minerals that are harder to get on even the best diet. Calcium, vitamin D, and other nutrients are commonly added to milks and cereals, and they are a great way to get what you might be missing.

Supplement With B12 and Vitamin D

Even omnivores are at risk of being deficient in vitamin B12 and vitamin D.

B12 naturally occurs in soil, is taken up by plants, and is then consumed by animals, where it is stored in their muscles. As our soils become more depleted, natural occurrence of B12 is starting to decrease so much so that even meat-eaters can be deficient.

There are currently no government recommendations for B12 supplement dosages for vegetarians. However, one study[22] suggests that doses of up to 6 micrograms of vitamin B12 per day may be appropriate for plant-based diets.

It is also more of a challenge getting enough vitamin D solely from plants. Many of the foods highest in vitamin D, such as salmon, egg yolks, and shellfish, aren't on the menu. But taking in sufficient amounts of vitamin D can be difficult on any diet, even for people who aren't vegan. One study found that 41.6 percent[23] of Americans may be deficient in vitamin D.

Plant-based sources include mushrooms and fortified milks, cereals, and orange juice.

Our bodies can create vitamin D from the sun, but as we tend to spend more and more time inside (or outside with sunscreen!), we often don't produce enough.

According to the National Institutes of Health24, an average daily intake of 400 to 800 IU, or 10 to 20 micrograms, is sufficient for more than 97 percent of people. Not all supplements are vegan, so be sure to check!

Don't Forget the Flavor!

Now that you have your basic plant-based plate design, it's time to spice it up! I like to choose a flavor profile first and then build my dish around that. One day it could be a Thai-inspired peanut sauce poured over vegetables, tofu, and rice. The next it could be a spicy tomato salsa topping bean and veggie burritos. Or it could be an Indian-style chickpea stew with carrots and onions over quinoa. The flavors of the world await!

Whole Foods That Fuel Runners Best

If you are anything like me, once you start to really get serious about becoming a better runner, you look to anything and everything that can help you become a better runner. You'll buy a foam roller and fancy socks and exotic powders all in the quest to be the best that you can be. But even if the latest running shoes can promise to make you 4 percent faster, it's the other 96 percent of you that matters most.

If you get the big stuff right, namely consistent training, good sleep, recovery, and nutrition, you will make the biggest impact on your running and race times. In this chapter, I'd like to get into the specifics of nutrition for runners, and specifically the vegetables that fuel you best and why.

The author Michael Pollen pretty much summed it up best by saying we should, "eat food, not too much, mostly plants."[25] And if you stick with that advice, you're doing a lot better than most. Whole, unprocessed food provides the most fiber and nutrients to our body and they are far harder to overeat than foods that have been so processed that they've done half the body's work for it. When building your meals, the best place to start is your vegetables. Your mom was right all along—you should eat your vegetables—and athletes need to eat more of them than sedentary folks. Half your plate should be non-starchy vegetables at every meal, and a quarter could be a starchy vegetable like potatoes if you are not in the mood for a whole grain.

Here's a breakdown of some awesome vegetables for runners and why they are so important.

Green Leafy Vegetables

Greens like kale are a good source of iron. If your diet is mostly or entirely plants, getting enough iron can be a challenge. Fortunately, dark green leaves are packed with iron, which is essential for preventing fatigue and iron deficiency anemia. Other plant sources of iron include watercress, chickpeas, lentils, beans, broccoli, and cabbage.

Spinach is another green that deserves a starring role on the table. Like other greens, spinach is a good source of vitamin B6, which is used to form hemoglobin in the blood. Hemoglobin helps red blood cells carry oxygen to your muscles, so if you're looking to boost your VO2 max, getting enough B6 can make a difference. Soybeans, chickpeas, lentils, other beans, and potatoes are other yummy sources.

My favorite way to eat greens is to fill a huge skillet with them and a few cloves of diced garlic. Pour in a little water to prevent them from sticking to the pan, and in a few short minutes, a massive pile of greens will wilt into a small cupful of garlicky goodness.

Broccoli

Broccoli is a good source of calcium. Calcium is the most commonly found mineral in the human body and is an essential electrolyte as well as a big factor in bone health. Strong bones are important for everyone, but especially runners that pound the pavement or the trails on the regular. Other vegetables high in calcium include cabbage, okra, and soybeans.

Sweet Potatoes

Sweet potatoes are a favorite food of mine, and they are a good source of beta-carotene. Turned into vitamin A by the body, beta-carotene plays a big role in supporting the immune system. So if you don't want to be sidelined with a cough or cold during training, try adding some beta-carotene with sweet potatoes or another orange-colored vegetable like squash or colored peppers. I love sweet potatoes roasted in the oven with just a touch of maple syrup and salt or mashed right out of the pressure cooker with a little chili powder and cumin.

Another B vitamin that is essential to get is B5, or pantothenic acid. It's found in tomatoes, mushrooms, avocados, and sunflower seeds. B5 helps you metabolize your food and turn it into the energy you need to run well.

Brussels Sprouts

Brussels sprouts are another mighty vegetable, and you might be surprised to learn that they are packed with vitamin C. Vitamin C is important for the immune system and healing injuries, and it's found in more than just citrus fruits. You'll get a nice dose of vitamin C in potatoes, broccoli, peppers, and cabbage. I prefer to roast brussels sprouts because it brings out a rich caramelized flavor so that the only seasoning needed is a light dusting of salt.

Legumes

Electrolytes such as potassium are key for maintaining a healthy balance of fluids in the body, essential for long distance runners. Most people know that bananas are a good source, but beans are even better. Chickpeas, lentils, and white beans are a great way of getting potassium into your diet without needing to resort to a sports drink. Other sources of potassium are mushrooms and beets.

Now some people would say that beans aren't a vegetable and that they are their own type of food, and that's certainly true—they are legumes. Beans are an inexpensive and important source of vitamins and minerals, such as folate, manganese, potassium, iron, copper, and magnesium. Not to mention they are a rich source of protein and carbohydrates.

As a runner, you need carbs to fuel your muscles and protein to build and repair your muscles, so a warm bowl of chili is a perfect way to refuel after a hard workout.

Beans are also high in fiber, which can help keep you full, keep you regular, and keep your gut microbiome healthy. A healthy gut means a strong immune system, which can keep you from getting sick.

Snacking on hummus with baby carrots, for example, contributes 8 to 10 grams of fiber towards the recommended daily target of 25 to 35 grams.

I can't mention every vegetable or legume that is good for you and why, but the good news is, there really isn't a vegetable that isn't good for you. So choose a wide variety of vegetables that you like, and be sure to „eat the rainbow," meaning pick vegetables that are all over the color spectrum to be sure that you are getting all the diverse nutrients that plants have to offer.

We runners tend to be the type to overcomplicate things, but when we get the basics right, like good training, good rest, and good nutrition, we can set ourselves up for our best running potential.

The Role of Starches in a Runner's Diet

What exactly is starch? Well, starch is a way that many plants store their extra glucose. Plants don't have a liver or muscles, so what they do is create banks of glucose that they can use later on for fuel. Well, at least until an animal or a human comes along and harvests that food bank for their self.

Starches are complex carbohydrates, which means they require digestion to be used by the body. Unlike simple sugar, which can be used quickly for fuel, starches need to be broken down into simple sugars first and therefore are absorbed more slowly.

Then there is something called resistant starch. Resistant starch naturally occurs in many whole foods, including cold rice, legumes, and unprocessed grains. The reason it's called resistant is because it resists digestion in your small intestine and must instead be broken down in your large intestine. And it's not just broken down into pieces. It actually ferments, which does all sorts of great things for your digestive health, not to mention it helps control blood sugar control and promotes the production of healthy fatty acids.

So what does all that mean for running?

Well, the reason I wanted to mention starch is because runners are constantly told to eat a high-carbohydrate diet for better performance, especially before running a marathon or participating in a hard workout. But to be honest, the word "carbohydrate" is a pretty terrible description of a huge class of foods. Lentils, lollipops, and lumber are all carbohydrates. Do you think your body processes them the same way? Of course not.

So it can be a lot more helpful to break that giant, all-encompassing word "carbohydrate" down into more useful categories. What some people use are the terms simple and complex to differentiate between so-called good and bad carbs.

The problem with that is that it's not so simple.

Most fruits, like watermelon, cherries, and grapes, as well as some vegetables, like carrots and beets, all contain simple carbohydrates, but they are also filled with fiber, nutrients, and phytochemicals that are great for human health. So using the terms simple and complex doesn't really help when you are deciding which carbs to put on your plate.

Okay, let's ditch simple and complex and use whole and refined. Now we're getting closer!

Refined foods are things like white rice, which has been stripped of the bran, white pasta, which has also been stripped of its bran and ground into flour, and basically anything made of refined flour or sugar, like many breads, cookies, and cupcakes.

So I could stop right there and say, "Just eat whole foods as much as possible and that would probably be way better than most of the diets out there." But for running performance, you want to be a little more refined than that. (See what I did there?)

Starchy foods include whole grains such as rice, quinoa, whole wheat, millet, oats, buckwheat, barley, and rye. Starchy vegetables include corn, potatoes, sweet potatoes, squash, pumpkins, beans, and peas.

Starchy whole foods are of course a good source of the energy you need to run well, but they are also a big source of a range of nutrients in our diet including fiber, calcium, iron, and B vitamins.

Some people think starchy foods are fattening, but gram for gram they contain fewer than half the calories of fat. For example, a tablespoon of oil has 120 calories, and it's one of the most concentrated sources of calories on the planet with virtually zero nutrients other than pure fat. Or you could eat a medium plain baked potato for 120 calories and you'd be getting fiber, vitamins B and C, iron, magnesium, potassium, and more. Not to mention you'll feel a lot fuller, with studies showing that they keep hunger away two to three times longer than other starches.

But don't just take my word for it if you think that carbs make you fat. In 2015, researchers at the University of South Carolina[26] had volunteers on a high-quality, high-carb vegan diet for six months. They lost an average of seven and a half percent of their initial body weight without making any attempts to eat less. One could argue that a whole foods plant-based diet is the key to weight management (I like that theory, of course). Or the takeaway here could be that when you replace low-quality, highly processed foods like pepperoni pizza and ice cream with whole foods, even if they are higher in carbohydrates, you can lose weight without eating less.

Beans are also an amazing starch for runners. Like potatoes, they are full of hunger-reducing fiber and resistant starch. Foods high in this resistant starch are shown to help promote weight loss because your body has to use extra energy to break them down. University of Colorado researchers found that adults who ate meals with resistant starch had higher postmeal metabolic rates. Resistant starches may also help control appetite.

Over and over again, scientific studies show that endurance athletes perform better with a higher carbohydrate intake, especially in the days leading up to a big race like a marathon.

But race-day performance is not always the focus in your everyday life, so the types of carbohydrates you choose to include on your make a difference in how you feel, how you look, and how you perform.

I feel like I've only scratched the surface here when it comes to starches, and I haven't even gotten to using starch as your fuel on race day instead of sugar! (See my UCAN recipe.)

Protein Is Not a Food, But You Still Have to Think About It

Order a salad in any restaurant and your enterprising, upselling server will inevitably ask you, "and what kind of protein would you like on that?" The rude answer that I tend to say in my head is, "Every plant food has protein! Stop believing it doesn't!"

While I've politely learned not to blurt out smarty-pants things to unsuspecting strangers, learning about the protein content of plant foods is important to everyone who is trying to add more nutrition to their plates.

Protein, along with fat and carbohydrate, is an essential macronutrient, not a food.

Sure, some foods contain a higher percentage of one macro over another, but we can't simply dissect the whole into its parts.

But we sure are fixated on trying, aren't we? If you wanted to, you could live like George Jetson and pop pills and powders and shakes to get your scientifically-approved, nutritionally optimal intake.

Yuck.

So with the exception of the Jetsons, we don't eat nutrients. We eat food.

How Much Protein Do I Really Need?

This is the age-old question, not just for athletes and herbivores, but for anyone.

The Recommended Daily Allowance (RDA) of protein for adults is 0.8 gram per kilogram of body weight. So for a 150-pound person, that's a scant 54 grams of protein a day.

You could eat a day's worth of calories from just white potatoes and get that much. I'm not suggesting you actually do that, but it's very easy to reach that goal from whole plant foods, provided that you are eating enough calories in general.

But is that really enough?

A recent meta-study referenced in the *New York Times* took a look at 49 high-quality past studies involving protein and muscle building in athletes and non-athletes. The authors found that everyone who strength trained gained muscle, no matter how much protein they ate.

Let me say that again: If you lift weights, you will gain muscle, with or without specifically paying attention to protein.

To me, this is the most important takeaway, because it means that you don't need to stress about guzzling protein shakes right after your workouts. But there's a difference between minimum requirements for protein and optimum. Because we're not just looking for the bare minimum; we want to know what's optimum for both health and athletic goals.

The authors of the study did find that those who increased their protein intake gained about 25 percent more muscle than those who only met the minimum. That's certainly significant enough to pay attention to.

As runners, we don't want huge muscle gains, but we do want to be strong and lean to run fast and stay injury free. This particular study indicates that 1.6 grams a day per kilo is ideal, but going higher than that has no muscular benefit.

That's important for the protein-shake people. Extra protein is simply extra calories your body doesn't need. So, if you're doing the math, there's a huge difference between the RDA of 0.8 gram per kilogram and the upper limit of 1.6 grams per kilogram.

Hey, that's double the RDA!

So our 150-pound runner is not going to get that kind of protein from the all-potato diet without significantly overeating (if it's even possible to eat 25 potatoes a day!). But by eating a variety of whole plant foods including nuts, seeds, legumes, and whole grains, it's not as hard as people think to reach the higher protein goals.

The good thing is that our protein intake can be spread out throughout the day since the researchers found no correlation between when you ate your protein or even what type of protein and how much muscle you gained.

But I'm a runner! I don't want to gain that much muscle.

Most runners want to gain nothing but speed. Weight gain, even the good muscular kind, feels a little scary since we equate it with being slow (which is not entirely true). In general, yes, most runners could stand to gain some muscle and lose some fat, but there is a point where too much muscle would be a problem. After all, The Rock has never won a marathon.

The thing to remember is protein intake is not the main driver of muscle building. It's lifting heavy things. So if you spend more of your time running than lifting, you'll end up with the body you need to run.

And with a few conscious choices about what you put on your plate, you can get all the protein you need to optimally (and deliciously) fuel your muscles.

No matter what the waiter thinks...

The Planted Runner Pantry

Just like a good night's sleep helps set you up for success in the morning, a well-stocked pantry can help you thrive in the kitchen. Plant-based cooking does not have to be complicated, time consuming, or expensive!

When you are first getting started, you might wonder how vegans can replicate the rich, savory flavor of cheese, the creaminess of dairy milk, or bake without eggs. I promise you, it's not only possible, but delicious! Of course, no plant can exactly replicate its animal counterpart in every case, but that's not always the goal. You can learn how to use plants in creative ways to satisfy your cravings without deprivation.

Put the "Veg" in Vegan

No matter what kind of diet is trending these days, vegetables are the undisputed superstars of a healthy diet. Full of fiber, nutrients, phytochemicals, water, vitamins, and minerals, vegetables should take up the biggest part of your plate. No longer relegated to side-dish status, veggies can take the starring role. Here are a few ideas:

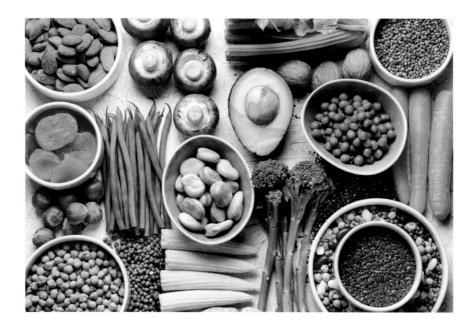

- Mushrooms can be grilled like steaks or chopped and browned to add a meaty flavor.
- Cauliflower coated with breadcrumbs and sauce makes incredible Buffalo bites.
- Shredded beets combined with beans and grains create savory red burgers.
- Butternut squash, roasted and seared, makes colorful chops that melt in your mouth.

When it comes to greens, you don't have to choose a sad side salad. Make your salad a hearty meal with chickpeas, carrots, red bell peppers, a scoop of quinoa, and a drizzle of balsamic vinaigrette.

My favorite way to eat greens isn't a salad, especially in the winter when I'm craving warm comfort food. I simply sauté some chopped onion and garlic in a little water, throw in a few huge handfuls of greens, and once wilted, sprinkle on some salt. It's amazing how an enormous amount of healthy greens will reduce into a satisfying, garlicky side dish!

Fantastic Fruit

Nutritionally rich and delicious, fruit is a key part of any runner's diet.

Bananas are probably the most ubiquitous runner's food. They are portable, full of simple-to-digest carbohydrates, and easy on the stomach. Many runners grab a banana pre-run to get quick fuel without worrying about it causing tummy trouble.

Tart cherries have recently been shown to help fight inflammation to better help you repair muscle damage from a hard workout.[3] You can drink tart cherry juice after a run or combine a handful of dried tart cherries with some mixed nuts for a great post-workout snack.

Berries of all kinds are crammed with antioxidants and phytochemicals which help promote recovery and boost the immune system. Add berries to smoothies or oatmeal or enjoy a bowl on its own for a sweet dessert.

Citrus fruits are filled with vitamin C which supports immune health. Vitamin C also helps the body absorb iron better, which can help runners who are at risk of anemia. Citrus fruits like oranges, tangerines, grapefruits, lemons, and limes are a flavorful and important addition to a runner's plate.

The Goodness of Grains

Grains can get an undeserved bad rap in some circles. Whole grains are a low-fat and affordable source of protein, vitamins, minerals, fiber, and nutrients. They can be the foundation of main dishes like a stir fry, burrito bowl, or salad, and they can add substance to burgers and soups.

There is a world of grains out there beyond wheat, rice, and corn. Barley, bulgar, farro, freekah, oats, and quinoa (technically a seed, but used as a grain) all have unique flavors, textures, and nutrient profiles that can add variety to your meals.

All grains go through some processing between cultivation and your plate, but you'll want to choose the least processed option as often as you can. White rice is more processed than brown rice, and wheat flour is more processed than wheat berries.

For products made with grain flours, like bread, look for the word "whole" at the top of the ingredients list to be sure that you are actually getting whole grains.

"Enriched" flour means that the grain was stripped of everything but the starch and then vitamins were added back in.

Lovely Legumes

The humble legume is a key player in a balanced plant-based diet. Beans, lentils, peanuts, peas, and soybeans are all inexpensive, versatile, protein-packed heroes.

Canned beans are convenient and easy to have on hand, but I prefer to cook dried beans in bulk in the pressure cooker. I portion out 2-cup servings into freezable mason jars so I always have a stash whenever I need them.

Lentils come in various shapes and sizes, and they are all quick-cooking and delicious. The brown and green kind can be found in any supermarket and add a meaty chew to tacos and pasta sauce. You might have to search the Indian section or grocery store for red lentils (which completely disappear when cooked, adding creaminess to curries and stews).

Edamame are young soybeans, typically left in their pods. When steamed and salted, they are the perfect nutty snack before a meal or after a run.

Chickpeas make the base for creamy hummus and add crunch and flavor to salads when dry roasted. They can also be mashed for a deli-style sandwich filling or smashed into savory falafel balls.

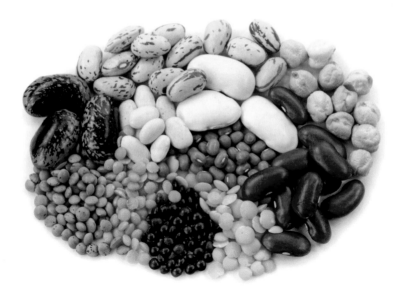

Green peas sometimes don't get the respect they deserve. These cute little protein balls can steal the spotlight on their own, pureed into a pesto, sprinkled in a soup, or chopped with walnuts, garlic, and salt into a chunky dip.

Super Soy

While beans and grains can provide runners with all the protein they need, there's no denying the incredibly rich protein power of soy.

Soy is a complete protein which means that it has adequate amounts of all the essential amino acids—the building blocks of protein. Soy has been grown and eaten in high quantities for thousands of years, primarily in Asia. Populations with diets high in soy protein and low in animal protein have lower risks of prostate and breast cancers. There has been a lot of conflicting information about soy and breast cancer over the past 25 years or so, with some people believing that soy is somehow harmful, yet the overwhelming evidence is that soy is safe and offers some preventative protection.[35]

Tofu, tempeh, and miso are the most widely available forms of soy products, and if prepared well, each are undeniably delicious. I admit, I was not a fan of tofu when I first went plant-based, but once I learned how to press the water out and sear it to perfection, I became hooked!

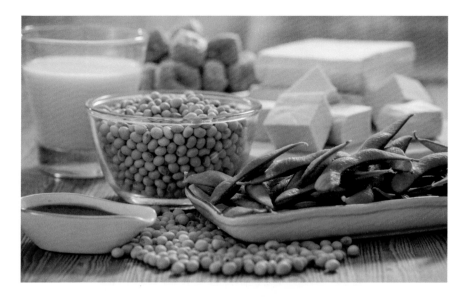

Nuts and Seeds

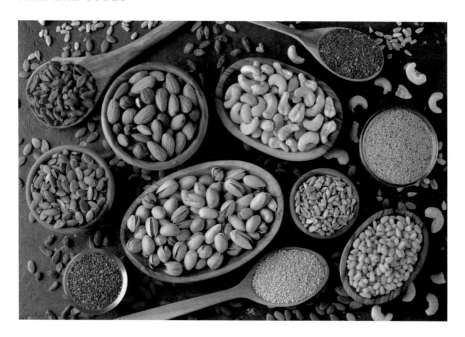

One of my go-to snacks after a sweaty run is a handful of salty mixed nuts and a fresh piece of fruit. But nuts don't have to be limited to snacks. They can be rich, creamy, or crunchy additions to your plant-based recipes.

Soaked cashews can be blended with sauteed onions, salt, and garlic to make a velvety alfredo sauce or a mozzarella-like topping for pizza.

Seeds like sesame, chia, flax, pumpkin, and sunflower might be tiny, but they are mighty sources of flavor, protein, and essential minerals. They are also a good whole food source of dietary fat, but a little goes a long way!

Plant-Based Milks

Plant-based milk options have exploded in recent years, and today, they dominate the dairy aisle. Soy, almond, oat, coconut, cashew, and flax are some of the many options. They all have slightly different tastes, uses, and flavor profiles, so experiment with what you like best.

You can even make your own at home from scratch, but store-bought milks are fortified with many of the vitamins and minerals that are harder to get on a vegan diet, like calcium and vitamin D.

Savor the Flavor

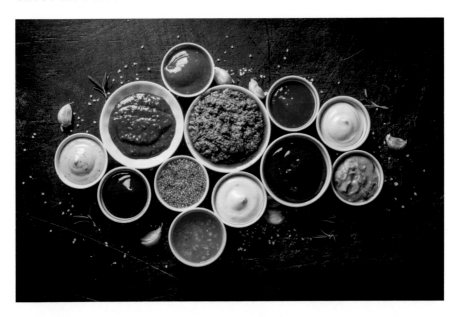

My biggest mistake when I first went plant-based was forgetting the flavor! I was trying so hard to make everything uber-healthy that nothing really tasted any good. Don't make the same mistake I did and focus on the flavor.

Herbs, spices, and good ol' salt and pepper can do wonders for any dish. But there are a few additions you'll want to add to your pantry to take your food to the next level of yummy:

- Soy sauce: This classic condiment gives food a salty, savory flavor known as umami. It can add depth to soups, sauces, and marinades.
- Tomato paste: The canned puree has a concentrated tomato flavor that adds richness to dips, spreads, and sauces
- Miso: Miso is made from fermented soybeans and is a welcome addition of umami for many recipes
- Nutritional yeast: Also known as "nooch," this dietary yeast has a nutty, cheesy flavor that can build depth and add a cheese-like bang anywhere you'd traditionally use cheese. As a bonus, it's naturally high in vitamin B12.
- Vinegar: Besides adding flavor, vinegar can be combined with baking soda to replace eggs in vegan cooking, as it helps baked goods bind together and rise.

My Favorite Cookbooks

I find myself reaching for the same cookbooks over and over again to prepare delicious, plant-based meals for my family. Here are some of my favorites:

Chloe's Kitchen, by Chloe Coscarelli. The first vegan to win TV's *Cupcake Wars*, all of Chloe's books make vegan cooking simple and delicious. Her first book, filled with fun recipes like cashew-based scalloped potatoes, pineapple fried rice, and amazing desserts, is still my favorite.

Forks Over Knives, The Cookbook, by Del Sroufe. From the same folks that brought us the groundbreaking documentary of the same name (and inspired my plant-based journey!), this classic cookbook has over 300 plant-based recipes that are tasty, simple, and affordable.

Vegan Richa's Indian Kitchen, by Richa Hingle. I love Indian cuisine, and making it at home is a lot less complicated than you might think! Easy-to-make restaurant-style dals, ruch curries, flatbreads, and savory treats at home.

Minimalist Baker's Everyday Cooking, by Dana Shultz. The powerhouse blogger's first book includes 101 entirely plant-based recipes that usually require minimal ingredients or dishes to clean. My favorites are the Vegan Caesar Salad and the Butternut Squash Mac 'n' Cheese.

This Cheese Is Nuts: Delicious Vegan Cheese at Home, by Julie Piatt. If the thought of missing cheese is enough to keep you from going entirely plant-based, this cookbook will change your mind. Ranging from a simple nacho sauce to a fermented cashew truffle cheese or a smoked gouda wheel, Julie shows us that no dairy cheese can't be made plant-based!

The Korean Vegan Cookbook: Reflections and Recipes from Omma's Kitchen, by Joanne Lee Molinaro. Beautifully photographed, this book is part cookbook and part family memoir. Learn how to make both traditional and reimagined Korean favorites in your own kitchen.

Chapter Two

Starting a Running Habit

Getting started with running fueled by plants and how walking can help you run faster and longer

The Run/Walk Method Is Great for Beginners (and Everyone Else)

When I started running again in my 20s, I thought the best plan for being able to run for a long time would be to just run as far as I could and then stop and walk back. I had no idea what I was doing and hadn't read a single thing on running but figured that my idea would work well enough to build up from couch to half marathon in a single summer (hey, I've always liked big goals!). The runs did get longer and longer, but wow, I spent a lot of time out there! My strategy did end up working, and I ran the half that fall, but there are probably better ways to incorporate a run/walk training plan that don't take up half your day.

When implemented correctly, a run/walk program is an effective training method that can help you increase your fitness level faster, recover from hard workouts quicker, and return from injury with less chance of relapse.

Let's start with the obvious place to begin: beginners.

The research says that aerobic development peaks between 30 to 90 minutes of exercise. You are building capillaries, increasing your plasma and blood volume, building up your heart and leg muscles and a whole lot more when you work out aerobically. But when you are just starting out, 30 minutes of running is far beyond most people's abilities.

That's when walking can take up the slack. You might start out with five minutes of brisk walking, then run for a few minutes, depending on your fitness level, and repeat. Your actual time spent running might only tally up to 10 or 15 minutes, but the time you are building your aerobic fitness level is far longer and hopefully pushes you into that 30- to 90-minute zone.

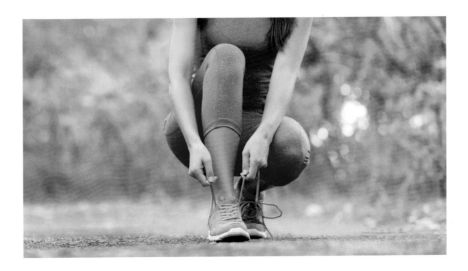

The walk breaks allow you to catch your breath, rest your legs a little, and stop the pounding that can be too much on your bones and tendons before they've had a chance to get used to it. That means you can get two to three times as much exercise (and calorie burn, if that's what you're after) in a far more gradual and gentler way, which allows you to progress faster than if you just run as long as you could all at once. (I wish I had known that in my 20s!)

You'll gradually want to increase your ratio of running to walking until you are doing all running. For example, if you started out with six minutes of running and four minutes of walking, you'll want to move up to seven minutes of running and three minutes of walking, and so on, eventually phasing out the walk altogether.

Once you build up to being able to get into the peak zone by just running, you might not need to keep up the walk part. The reason for this is because at a certain level of fitness, walking is not going to give you the same stimulus as just running. Once a 30- to 45-minute run feels easy without walk breaks, your running will progress faster without the walks, in general.

One exception is your long run. If you are trying to build that up, a good strategy is to keep a walk in there, even if you are running 30 to 45 minutes on your weekday runs without stopping. For example, you might do 20 minutes of running with 2 minutes of walking three times for a total of 64 minutes on the weekend. By keeping the walk in there for three to four weeks on your long run, you can be sure that you are not overstressing your body and are better prepared for the distance.

But once you are ready to drop the walk during your runs, that doesn't mean that you should stop walking! Walking is one of the best cross training activities because it's easy, gentle, free, and very similar to running. Instead of a pure rest day after a hard day of running, you might want to try a 30-minute walk. You will likely recover better and boost your aerobic fitness level and metabolism at the same time. And that is something that every kind of runner can benefit from.

Experienced runners sometimes suffer from a stubborn belief that only running will make them better runners, and that's simply not true. Walk breaks can help make a recovery run feel better and be less stressful on the skeletal system, so don't let your ego stop you from taking a beneficial walk break on a particularly junky-feeling Wednesday run.

The low-stress benefits of the run/walk are also the best way to return to running from injury or a significant break in training for whatever reason. If you had to stop running for more than two weeks, or the injury is particularly difficult, the run walk method can prevent re-injury and help you transition back to normal training faster than running alone.

Now, I know what the veteran runners are thinking here, and you might be saying something like, "I've been running for years, why on earth do I need to start walking every 10 minutes coming back from my hamstring injury? I'm in a hurry to get back to training because my goal race is just around the corner and this walking business is such a waste of time. Certainly not for me!"

Well, actually, if you're in a hurry, this might be the faster road to recovery, as counterintuitive as that may seem. That's because when returning from a difficult or persistent injury, the injured area is likely to be sensitive and prone to re-injury.

When we hurry back to running, we tend to ignore the mild to moderate pain signals, which causes the body to compensate for the injury by changing how you run to lessen the pain. This could be an obvious limp, or it could be completely invisible as the body shifts the pressure from the injured area to another muscle group that is not prepared to handle the load.

This means that you could potentially be stressing other areas of your body to compensate and set off a chain of injuries. This is why sprained ankles lead to iliotibial (IT) band and knee pain and strained hamstrings might lead to calf trouble.

Not ideal.

But by implementing a run/walk, you will help take pressure off your structural system while enabling you to get out and run for a greater total time while transitioning back to normal training.

If your ego is still getting in the way of a walk, it might help to know that top elites will utilize the run/walk method when coming back from injury, and running is their job! Their egos and their livelihoods are invested in getting back to running as fast as possible, and often, the best way to do that is to walk.

So if you've been injured and you are back to running, but progress is slow and pain is still there, try breaking up the run with some walking for a couple of weeks and see how it goes.

Human beings were designed to walk a lot more than most of us actually do, and by incorporating more walking in our lives, we all can become better runners.

The Importance of Warm-Ups and Cool-Downs

Most runners know that they should not just get out of bed and start sprinting right away. And most runners also know that they should probably do some kind of cool-down at the end of their runs as well.

But let's face it. When we are short on time, the warm-up and cool-down is the first to get axed, right? We are runners, and we just want to run!

But what if I told you that by skipping the warm-up and cool-down, you are actually doing your running a disservice? Properly warming up and cooling down can make you a faster and less injury-prone runner, even if it means you have to cut some of your mileage to fit it all in.

Let's first talk about the warm-up. Most runners think a mile or two of easy jogging is good enough for a warm-up before a workout. And that might be true, but somewhere around 30 to 70 percent of runners get injured every year, so you might not want to automatically trust what most runners are doing.

What a warm-up does is two things. First, it slowly prepares your body for the work you are about to do, literally warming up your muscles by circulating your blood.

Your heart rate gently rises, and your breathing also gently increases. By the time you are ready for your faster paced running, your body is up to speed, and it's not as much of a shock.

Have you ever run up a flight or two of stairs only to find yourself out of breath at the top? You might say to yourself, "Hey, I'm a marathon runner! Why on earth am I out of breath after climbing a flight of stairs?" The answer is that you were not warmed up. When you go from a full stop to top speed, your circulatory system is not yet fully engaged, and the effort will feel much harder than if you have eased into it.

The second thing a warm-up does is build and reinforce the communication pathways between the brain and the muscles. These are called neuromuscular connections. Your running form, efficiency, economy, power, stride length, stride frequency, and, ultimately, fatigue resistance are all neuromuscular in nature. None of them will be developed just by focusing on jogging an easy warm-up mile.

Neuromuscular training is about stimulating the brain's communication with the muscles. To do that, we use specific drills that involve an element of concentration and a little bit of skill. Remember, we are trying to stimulate the brain and encourage it to communicate and activate more muscle fibers more quickly, with the goal of improving the efficiency of each stride. Simply going through the motions is not enough.

There are several classic drills that you can use in a dynamic warm-up, and they should only take 5 to 10 minutes. The lunge matrix, or doing several lunges on each leg forwards, backwards, and to the side is a great place to start. You can check out how to do those on YouTube by searching for "Jay Johnson lunge matrix."

One of my favorite drills is leg swings. Find something to hold on to for balance, and swing your leg forwards and backwards 8 to 10 times, then do it side to side and switch legs. This helps with your hip extension as well as focuses on lateral mobility. If you want to get your core involved a bit more, try doing them without holding on to anything.

There are about a million more warm-up drills that you can use, and what you choose should be tailored to the areas that you need to work on. For example, if you have IT band issues, you should include hip drops. If you need more glute activation, you could try donkey kicks or squat thrusts to wake up these areas.

When you incorporate drills as an essential part of your warm-up, you are getting more bang for your running buck, so don't skip them!

What about the cool-down? What's so important about that?

The goal of performing a cool-down and recovery routine is to return the body back to its resting state as efficiently as possible, flush out the waste products you've built up on the run, and maintain healthy muscle function. Doing so prompts quick and complete recovery in preparation for the next hard effort. Stopping abruptly after runs encourages blood pooling and can cause dizziness, so you want to make the transition gentle.

While your cool-down should be easy enough that you won't create much additional waste, your heart rate will stay sufficiently raised to send the healing and recovering effect of your circulatory system to work. Blood clears out metabolic waste and hormones while proteins and white blood cells begin healing microtears in the muscles.

For most faster runners, you can cool down with some light jogging. If you are a slower runner, a brisk walk is a better choice.

The length of your cool-down depends on what you just ran. If it was a short, easy run, ending with some jogging or walking for a few minutes is great. Finish up with five to six minutes of foam rolling and dynamic stretching, and you're good to go.

If you had a hard workout, you'll want to extend the cool-down a bit more and be sure that you are getting an extra few minutes on the roller for your full body.

For a long run or a big race, you want to jog your cool-down, but you might want to wait a few hours for the roller or stretching. Your muscles need time to get blood and nutrients to them after a big effort, and foam rolling or massage immediately on damaged muscles is not ideal.

Post run is a great time to include some of the active isolated stretching (AIS) exercises that I talked about earlier. Not only do they feel really good after a run, but you also get to lie down on the floor, which is perfect when you are tired from a good run!

I hope this helps reinforce the importance of a good warm-up and cool-down. When you are short on time, cut a little of your workout time instead of the warm-up or cool-down, even though that might seem counterintuitive. Your body will thank you.

Run Slower to Get Faster

It seems paradoxical, but running slower most of the time will make you a faster runner. You see, building peak aerobic fitness takes a very long time, years and years actually, so the slower the aerobic work you do every week, the earlier the results you are looking for will come.

So how exactly do you run slow? And how slow is slow? I'll get to that part in the section, The Art of Running Slow.

How Slow Running Can Make You Faster

I know it sounds counterintuitive that slow running will make you faster, but it's true. Convincing my athletes to slow down their easy runs is often the hardest thing I do as a coach!

What most uncoached runners do is just go out for a run at whatever pace feels good. Most of the time, they run too fast. I mean, we runners love to see progress, and it makes sense that if our normal, everyday run gets faster, we must be getting faster, too, right?

Well, what's actually happening is that most people are just running in their happy middle zone most of the time. It's not so fast that it's hard or really challenging, but not so slow that people would call it "jogging." Heaven forbid!

But as crazy as it sounds, the secret to speeding up is slowing down. That's right, I'm telling you to move your ego aside most of the time and embrace the jog. Become friends with the jog. Take the word "jog" back, and declare yourself a jogger, loud and proud. And then go crush your PRs.

How can this be?

The easiest way to explain it is that the more running you do, the better a runner you will become up to a point. A little high-intensity speedwork goes a long way, and results are seen quickly, but just a little too much speed, and your risk of injury and overtraining goes up dramatically while the return on your running investment goes way down. So by keeping about 80 percent of your running slow, you build a big aerobic engine with a much lower risk.

Another way to picture it is that slow running is the cake, and fast running is the icing. You could eat a lot of unfrosted cake, but it's pretty hard to eat a giant bowl of just frosting. But get the ratio right, and you have a perfect dessert.

Let's look at the science behind the theory, and then I'll explain exactly how you can run slow enough to become faster.

Slow Running Boosts the Aerobic System

One of the primary reasons to run slowly on your easy days and for most of your long runs is that slower running builds the aerobic system. In order to exercise, your body needs to break down carbohydrate and convert it to glycogen so it can be used as energy or fuel.

With enough oxygen, the body will use the aerobic system, also known as aerobic glycolysis, to create energy, or ATP, to power endurance running.

When you breathe in, IF you are going slow enough, the body efficiently uses all the oxygen it needs to power the muscles, and then you exhale.

As you continue to run aerobically over time, your body gets better and better at using oxygen to make energy, which allows you to run faster when you want to.

And the reason having a great aerobic system is critical is because 85 to 99 percent of the energy needed to race any distance longer than 800 meters comes from the aerobic system.

There is simply no better way to train the aerobic system than easy running.

Capillary and Mitochondria Development

These are the two major physiological developments that occur with aerobic training. (There are several more, but let's not get too bogged down in the science for now!)

Capillaries are tiny blood vessels, and they help bring oxygen and nutrients to the muscle tissues while taking waste products out. The more capillaries you have surrounding each muscle fiber, the faster you can transport oxygen and carbohydrate into your muscles.

Aerobic training, by running easy, increases the number of capillaries per muscle fiber. This means your muscles get more oxygen and nutrients while waste products are removed faster. With more oxygen and less waste, you can run faster.

Mitochondria are microscopic organelle found in your muscles' cells that contribute to the production of ATP (energy). The job of mitochondria is to break down carbohydrate, fat, and protein into usable energy, if there's enough oxygen around.

The more mitochondria you have, and the greater their density, the more energy you can generate during exercise. That will enable you to run faster and longer! Aerobic training increases both the number and the size of the mitochondria in your muscle fibers.

Running Faster Isn't as Aerobically Effective

Okay, so we know that building the aerobic system allows us to run faster, but doesn't it make more sense to make that happen faster by running faster every day?

Unfortunately, it doesn't work that way. Not only will running faster result in diminished aerobic development, but it increases the chances of injury and overtraining. Let's look at why.

Scientific research has shown that peak capillary development happens between 60 and 75 percent of 5k pace. Faster running may actually inhibit the process. And maximum mitochondrial development occurs when running at 55 to 75 percent of 5k pace.

In other words, the optimal easy run pace for aerobic development is between 55 and 75 percent of your 5k pace. That is going to feel VERY slow if you are not used to it. For a 20-minute 5k runner, that's somewhere around 9:45 pace. For a 30-minute 5k runner, that's more like 12- to 13-minute pace.

If you don't know your 5k race pace, that's okay. Actual pacing on an easy run doesn't have to be that complicated! More on that in just a minute.

But What If I'm Feeling Good and Want to Run Faster?

While the science is absolutely clear that running faster isn't going to develop your aerobic system more rapidly, many runners wonder, what's the harm in running faster on those days you feel good? The problem with that is the faster you run on your easy days, the more stress you place on the muscles, tendons, ligaments, and bones.

On days where you are feeling fresh, it's fun to go faster. But if your hips aren't strong enough yet to handle the pace or the extra days of faster running, it wouldn't be surprising if your IT band becomes inflamed or your hamstring gets angry.

Even if your breathing is fine, you are setting yourself up for injury.

Slow Running Promotes Recovery From Faster Running

Besides building a big aerobic engine, easy days can help you recover from your hard workouts and run those speed days faster– but not if you run your easy days too fast.

After a speedy workout, your muscles will have micro-tears from the forceful contractions that happen at fast speeds. These micro-tears cause muscle soreness and make training the day after a hard workout extra hard. The body heals these small micro-tears through the circulatory system, delivering oxygen and nutrients to the muscles that need repair.

When you run easy, oxygen and nutrients are delivered directly to the muscles used during running. That is why an easy run might be more beneficial than a complete rest day. If you run easy enough, the stress and micro-tears that result from running are virtually non-existent. In other words, you don't need a recovery day from your recovery run.

The Art of Running Slowly

By now, I hope I've convinced you with the science to slow down those easy runs. So how exactly do you do it?

Anytime you are doing something you are not used to, it will feel awkward, and running slowly is no exception. If you are used to running at a moderate pace, your body will complain when you try to change that, but I promise you, it will get easier.

So here's how you do it, and once again, it's simple, but it might not be easy. Your form shouldn't change much at all. You just shorten your stride. You should still keep a nice, quick cadence and good posture with your head up and your shoulders down away from your ears. You want to be light and smooth on your feet, and never be double supported, meaning no shuffling! One foot on the ground at a time. You want to be like a quiet little ninja. So quiet that you sneak up on people ahead of you and scare the daylights out of them as you pass by.

One trick to being sure you are running easy is to close your mouth. If you can run breathing only out of your nose, then you are running easy! Now I'm not saying that you have to nose breathe the whole time, but it's just a little test if you are by yourself.

If you are running with a friend, use the talk test. You should be able to carry on a full conversation with your running buddy just as easily as you could while walking.

When you run slowly, you are not only building your aerobic engine so that you can race faster and longer, but you are also moving nutrients to your hard-working muscles so they can repair and build from your faster speed days. By the time your next hard session comes along, you are fresh and recovered, ready to run harder than you would be able to if you were still sore.

And what that means is that you are maximizing the short time that you run fast each week, which will get you faster, faster.

There really is no such thing as too slow on an easy day as long as you are not just out there shuffling. You are still hopping from one foot to the next with each step.

The pace of your slow run will vary depending on your fitness level, but a good rule of thumb is that you should be going at least one minute per mile slower than your marathon pace, and two minutes is probably even better. For you really fast folks out there, you could even be going three minutes slower. The thing is, you really can't go too slow on your slow days. It might not seem like it, but you are getting results.

Now, many of my coaching clients will say to me, "I can't run that slow! My form completely breaks down when I run slowly, and it feels awkward and uncomfortable."

Notice that I have been using the word "slow" and not the word "easy." Slow and easy are not the same thing. Let go of any thoughts of easy, hard, comfortable, and so on. Some days slow runs will feel easy, and other days, like when you are sore after a tough workout the day before, they will not feel easy at all.

But they should always feel slow.

Once you get the physical form of running easy down, the next thing to do is make sure your ego is on board. Running slowly can feel somehow embarrassing, even though it shouldn't. It's a necessary part of training and should be done with purpose and pride.

Confidence in your running ability will come when you train smart and see the results of your hard work. It takes patience, but it's well worth the effort. If you'd like to not only run faster, but remain a runner for life, easy running, about 80 percent of the time, is the most effective way to get there.

How to Gauge Your Effort

If you are new to running, you might want to know how hard you should be working every day. Let's face it, even if you've been running for years, you might still not know exactly how hard your runs should feel.

And with today's technology, you might think that you really don't have to. Most of us are wearing a powerful computer on our wrists or in our phones, and the data can be crunched and analyzed and computed for us. It can tell us how hard we are working, how fit we are, how much sleep we need, and how long we should recover.

But the truth is, all that quantification is only a rough guess, no matter how science-like it looks. How fast you got from point A to point B is a fact, but how you felt getting there will tell you a lot more than any watch can.

Here's a Rating of Perceived Effort (RPE) scale that can help.

And remember, this is a scale of running effort, so walking or sitting on the couch are off the chart, effectively being a zero, even though obviously you need to spend a little effort to get up off that couch and go for a walk. So unless you are a race walker, walking effort is not included.

Your hard days should most often be in the seven to eight range and occasionally (but rarely) a nine. Easy days should be between one and three.

HOW SHOULD YOUR RUNS *feel?*

the planted runner

1	**Slow, relaxed jogging. Just barely more difficult than a walk**
2	**Still gentle and easy running. Can hold a conversation or sing aloud to music**
3	**Breathing is a little heavier, but you can still carry on a shorter conversation most of the run**
4	**Effort is noticeable, you are breathing harder, but can still say several full sentences in a row**
5	**Medium effort run, harder breathing, but not gasping. You can talk but you need to concentrate**
6	**Comfortably hard, heavy breathing, talking is not fun, but you can say a sentence if you have to**
7	**Challenging, but doable. Heavy concentration needed to maintain effort. Can say a short sentence**
8	**Very hard, yet not all-out. Very heavy breathing, can only blurt out a couple of words at a time**
9	**Very hard to maintain. Very hard to breathe. Talking is nearly impossible**
10	**Unsustainable, all-out, chased-by-a-tiger effort**

Hanging out in the medium effort zone is something that should be pretty rare. It can be done occasionally the day before a hard long run to better simulate race day fatigue, or you might consider a long slow easy run to be a medium effort simply because of the distance. But the cycle of stimulus and recovery is best achieved with polarized training, so you want to stay on the ends of the scale most of the time.

Running by effort is not always an intuitive thing, but you will get better at it. Knowing why you are running at a certain effort level also helps you achieve your goals better because you are running with purpose.

Now I'm not suggesting that you throw away your watch and start running based on whatever mood you happen to be in. Not at all. But figuring out a system of being able to communicate to yourself and your coach how hard a run was is more important than whatever the numbers on the watch say.

Chapter Three

Fueling Your Runs

Learn what to eat and when to fuel your best running life

The Best Foods to Eat Before a Run

If you are an early morning runner, you probably head out the door as soon as your shoes are tied. There's no time to eat a meal, wait for it to digest, contemplate why you got up so crazy early in the morning when the rest of the world is peacefully sleeping...and then go for your run.

But there are benefits to eating before a run, even very early in the morning, so now I'd like to go over exactly what you should eat before you head out the door, no matter what kind of run you plan to do or what time of day it is.

Do You HAVE to Eat Before a Run?

Before we talk about what you should eat to fuel your run, let's start with whether or not you need to eat anything at all. Millions of runners wake up every day and head out for their run completely fasted, or quite literally running on empty.

Many would argue that you don't need any fuel at all for a normal, easy run that is less than 60 minutes. After all, you have plenty of stored glycogen in your muscles and a virtually unlimited supply of fat that will get you through an easy run. While that is true, it is still a good idea to put something in the tank, even if it's early in the morning.

Sports dietician Meghann Featherstunn is passionate about the reasons why all runners should fuel, especially if they are training hard for a big race. And that includes fueling for your easy runs as well:

"I highly, highly, highly recommend that before any run you are eating something," she said when we spoke in 2021. "When we are waking up and working out immediately in the morning, that's when it's most important to eat. Our body is in a catabolic state where muscle is breaking down, then we go for a run and break it down even more. We have had this prolonged state of our body breaking itself down. There's some really great research out there that this is terrible for our hormones. We are in this major caloric hole and our bodies hate that."

What Foods Are Best?

So it's pretty clear that we do need to eat before we run, but what types of foods should we choose?

When trying to figure out what you should eat to fuel your run, the first thing you need to determine is what kind of run you are about to have. An easy 30-minute jog is going to have different fuel requirements than a long run, marathon, or hard speed session.

I'll go over the differences in more detail shortly, but unless you are running very slowly for a very long period, what all your runs have in common is that carbohydrate-rich foods will help fuel you the best.

Many health-conscious runners get a little worried when I tell them to eat simple carbohydrates, but remember, you are not about to sit on the couch! You are fueling for performance and everything you eat will be used for fuel, not stored as fat.

Even with experts like Meghann practically begging runners to eat something before a run, it can be tough to do, especially if you have a sensitive stomach. The best way to deal with that is to experiment with very small amounts of foods that are quick to grab and easy to digest until you find out what works for you right out the door.

And once you find it, make sure that you always have it in the house ready to go.

Quick Carbs

What makes a perfect pre-run food? Something that is high in carbohydrate and low in just about everything else like protein, fat, and fiber.

For an easy run first thing in the morning, try starting with a half a banana, a fig bar, or a date. Maybe grab a handful of Cheerios or munch on a couple of Saltine crackers. Some runners do well with fruit juice or applesauce, while others find the fructose hard on their stomachs.

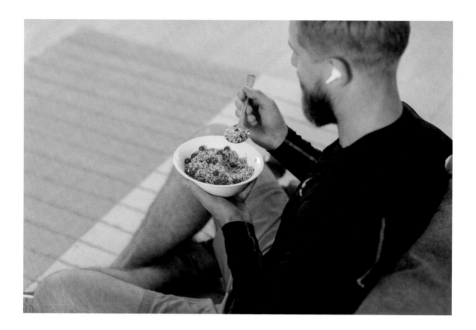

Meghann's favorite choice is a graham cracker or two or a simple white bagel. Again, the trick is to start very small and build with each run, because just like your muscles, the stomach can be trained. Morning runners might have to try getting up a few minutes earlier, but it will be worth it when the day comes when you can truly eat and run.

If you are running a shorter easy run at a different time of day, there's no need for extra fuel if you've eaten in the last one to three hours.

Fuel for Long or Fast Runs

As you start to plan your fueling for longer and faster running, the equations will look a little different. As I mentioned earlier, what you eat and when you eat it before a run will depend on when you ate last and the type of run you are about to do. The tougher or longer the run, the more important it is to get both the timing and the food just right.

Like most aspects of training, finding the optimal time to eat before a run is an individual preference. But in general, the harder you have to run, the earlier and more substantially you should eat. This is to ensure that you not only have enough fuel on board but that you don't have a lot in your stomach, which can cause issues.

Now there are some runners that can eat just about anything within 30 minutes before a run and they are good to go. If that's you, you're amazing. But if you are like most runners, you'll need to play with the timing to figure out what's best for you.

A good rule of thumb is if you have a long run or workout that is going to take more than 90 minutes to complete, you will need extra fuel. Yes, it's true that you have about two hours of fuel stored in your muscles and liver, but your brain will start to protest by slowing you down long before the two-hour mark.

Snacks or Mini-Meals

I recommend trying to eat a medium sized snack or a mini-meal about 90 minutes before your hard run. The exact calorie counts will look different for every runner, but it could be roughly in the 200 to 400 calorie range.

That could be a bagel with hummus, a small peanut butter and jelly sandwich, or even something super simple like a bowl of rice with soy sauce for sodium and flavor, maybe with a drizzle of tahini or a few slices of avocado for a little extra staying power. A classic long-run breakfast is oatmeal with maple syrup with maybe a few blueberries sprinkled on top.

As you might have noticed, these mini-meals are not entirely carbohydrates. They also have a little fat and protein to help keep you from being hungry again right as you start the run.

Many runners turn to commercial bars, gels, and powders for pre-run foods, and if you like the convenience of those, there's not really anything wrong with that because you will burn it all off in your run. But in general, I'd say save the specialty products for the run itself and eat whole foods before and after.

Trial and Error

Now, if you've tried fueling before a hard run before and you just can't stomach it, remember that the stomach can be trained, but you will have to experiment.

- Start with a small snack two hours ahead of your hard or long run.
- If your stomach handles it well, next time try moving the same snack forward 15 to 20 minutes.

- But, if you experience stomach issues, push back the timing of your snack 15 to 20 minutes, and maybe tweak the recipe a bit.
- Keep moving forward or backward 15 to 20 minutes per run until you find the closest time you can eat before you have any issues. This way, you'll know exactly what foods sit well with you and exactly when to eat them on important workout days and race day.

These are just some sample ideas of what you can eat before a run to stay energized and prevent stomach issues. While eating before a run is highly individualized, with a few simple experiments, you can find the optimal pre-run meal or snack for you, even if you run first thing in the morning.

By fueling properly and not eating too little or too much before you head out for your long training runs, you can maximize your training and start seeing results sooner.

Glycogen Metabolism

Let's dive a little deeper into how your body uses, stores, and burns fuel to create energy.

When you run, active muscle cells require a constant supply of energy in the form of a molecule called ATP. ATP is made by oxidizing fat, which comes from fatty acids in the bloodstream or triglyceride stored in the muscle along with glucose supplied by the bloodstream and the glycogen stored in the muscle.

In other words, your body makes the molecule needed for energy from fat and sugar, which is supplied to the muscle cells either from the blood or from stores in the muscle itself.

When you exercise, you are never only burning glycogen. You burn fat as well, but the ratio is different at different intensities and depends on how adept your body is at burning fat and what you ate for breakfast. For now, let's focus on glycogen, because although muscle and liver glycogen represent just four percent of the body's total fuel stores, muscle glycogen is the primary fuel during exercise of moderate or greater intensity.

But first of all, what is it?

In the human body, glycogen is a particle made up of individual glucose molecules. About 20 percent is stored in the liver, and around 80 percent is in your skeletal muscle. (Glycogen is also present in small amounts in other tissues, but to keep this simple, let's not get into all of that right now.)

The more muscle mass you have, the greater the amount of glycogen that can be stored, and the fitter you are, the better the entire process works. Most people have somewhere around 1400 to 2000 calories' worth of glycogen stored in fully fueled muscles or about 350 to 500 grams. In the liver, you'll have somewhere around 100 grams or 400 calories stored.

The glycogen in your liver is used mainly to fuel the normal functioning of the body and the brain, while the glycogen stored in your muscles is conveniently located to fuel the muscle itself. The glucose stored as liver glycogen is used to constantly keep a stable level of glucose circulating in your blood. To ensure the brain has an ample supply of glucose, the liver releases glucose into the bloodstream at about the same rate as it is used by the tissues, creating a nice balance of supply and demand.

Your hungry brain is the biggest consumer of blood glucose. Under normal circumstances, glucose is the only fuel the brain uses. At rest, approximately 60 percent of the glucose found in blood is metabolized by the brain.

When liver glycogen stores fall to low levels, the liver can make its own glucose from things like amino acids (aka protein) but this process is limited and cannot keep pace with the demand for glucose during a hard or long run. So instead, your body starts to tap into a rich source of glycogen, and that's in your muscles.

Remember, your body's number one priority is to feed that big brain, not go running for four hours. So when your liver gets low on fuel, it will steal it from the muscles, which at some point will slow you down. But if you keep the supply of glucose coming while you are working out, your storage tanks stay full in both the liver and the muscles, and everyone's happy.

Up to a certain point, of course.

How is glycogen created? Two ways: The body makes it directly from the food we eat or creates it through a process called gluconeogenesis using things like the lactate that you built up when you ran hard.

Glycogen is accumulated in the liver primarily after eating and buildup in the skeletal muscle occurs mainly after exercise, especially in athletes. This means that after a run, the carbohydrate you eat replenishes your muscles' fuel so that you can run well again the next day. When you sprint hard or run long, muscle glycogen particles are broken down. This frees glucose molecules that muscle cells then oxidize either anaerobically or aerobically.

The rate at which muscle glycogen is broken down and depleted depends primarily upon the intensity of the run. The harder you run, the faster the muscle glycogen is broken down. That means intervals and hill repeats are going to lower your glycogen stores in the active muscle cells at a faster rate than would an easy long run.

The good news for runners is that the more fit you are, the bigger your storage tanks get. As you run longer and longer, your glycogen stores are reduced, and fatty acids in the blood become more available. Endurance training not only increases muscle glycogen stores but also reduces the reliance on glycogen because those free fatty acids are more ready for use by active muscle cells. In other words, you become more fat-adapted simply by endurance training, without having to go paleo.

Replenishing your glycogen stores after a long or hard workout is an important part of the recovery process and will get you ready to run hard again sooner. Your body hates having a low balance in the glycogen bank account and will do everything it can to stock up, even if it means cannibalizing the protein in your muscles to do it. Not only is losing muscle a bad thing, but it hurts! Soreness, fatigue, or just feeling a bit off can all be signs that your body wants a carbohydrate deposit as soon as possible. So grab that banana when you are done.

I have just scratched the surface when it comes to the science behind the body's use of glycogen. But the reality is that it's pretty simple. Train smart and often, eat a balanced, whole foods diet rich in fruits, vegetables, and grains, and don't forget to eat after your hard runs.

The 411 on 4:1 Ratios for Recovery

When we go for a hard run or lift weights at the gym, we are not building our muscles. We are breaking them down. Muscles grow when they repair, and fueling your body properly after a workout will give your body all it needs to recover and grow stronger.

If a run is more than 60 minutes long, your body is primed for recovery[27] as soon as you stop.

Most exercise science research says that the ideal window to eat after a hard workout is 30 to 60 minutes because your body is ready to begin the muscle repair process instead of the fat storage process, but the thing to remember is that your body isn't stupid. It will use the tools you give it to repair your muscles whether you are in that perfect window or not, so you don't have to guzzle down a protein shake at the gym because you are afraid you are going to miss some magical repair moment. You can go home and eat real food instead.

Ideally, you should aim to time your workout to end before a mealtime so that you eat something balanced and substantial instead of just a snack. Eating a small snack after a workout is fine in a pinch, but if you have really depleted your body's glycogen stores on a long or hard run, your best bet is a real meal.

So if you like to work out in the morning, have breakfast or lunch after you work out. If you are an afternoon runner, eat dinner after you run.

The things your body needs, whether you ran hard or lifted hard, are carbohydrate and protein. Healthy fat is essential for good health, too, but it's relatively easy to get and should not be your main focus.

And contrary to popular belief, you do not need huge amounts of recovery protein after lifting weights. The body uses only about 20 to 30 grams of protein at one time to build muscle. That's typically less than the average hungry athlete eats.

If you can't time your workout to end at a mealtime, or if you didn't work out very hard for you, maybe all you need is a small snack, somewhere in the 200 to 300 calorie range. For this type of snack, I recommend skipping the bars and the shakes and going for fruit with nuts. So a banana with peanut butter or an apple with a small handful of walnuts or a nice trail mix blend of dried fruit and nuts. You don't want to go overboard because you'll be eating a meal in a couple of hours, so consume just enough to tide you over.

There are plenty of sports nutrition companies out there ready to fill that need and take your money. Some are great whole food choices (Picky Bars, Lara Bars), and some are full of unpronounceable ingredients. But is it really necessary or important to eat an expensive bar or blend a multi-ingredient kale smoothie with a scoop of expensive protein powder to get the best recovery?

Nope. This might sound shocking, but you can **just eat real food**. It's true.

What kind of food? The science says the best way to replenish your glycogen and begin the muscle repair process is to fuel yourself with carbs and a small amount of protein. Some claim the ratio should be four grams of carbs to one gram of protein, others say it's 3:1, and others are somewhere in between[28]. In fact, the exact ratio might not matter so much as long as you are getting some of each.

Here are some great combos of whole foods that are great for recovery after **shorter runs**.

- A medium apple with 2 tablespoons of natural peanut butter: 270 calories, 24 grams carbs, 8 grams protein, **ratio of 3**
- 25 almonds and 4 unsulfured dried apricots: 216 calories, 24.6 grams carbs, 5.7 grams protein, **ratio of 4.34**
- 4 tablespoons hummus, 12 baby carrots: 203 calories, 22.8 grams carbs, 5.2 grams protein, **ratio of 4.3**
- 1/2 cup chickpeas: 134 calories, 22.5 grams carbs, 7.5 grams protein, **ratio of 3**
- 1/2 cup jasmine rice, 2/3 cup green peas (add some soy sauce for salt and flavor): 210 calories, 24.5 grams carbs, 8 grams protein, **ratio of 3.06**
- 1 medjool date and 1 ounce (1/4 cup) of cashews: 226 calories, 26.5 grams carbs, 5.7 grams protein, **ratio of 4.6**
- Banana with 2 tablespoons almond butter: 290 calories, 29 grams carbs, 8.3 grams protein, **ratio of 3.49**
- 2.5 cups kale and 1/2 a white onion, sauteed in vegetable broth, with 1/2 cup white beans: 201 calories, 39 grams carbs, 11.8 grams protein, **ratio of 3.3** (love this for lots of volume without too many calories!)

If you can time your run to end right before a meal, your meal will be your recovery fuel. This is a great tool in avoiding too much snacking if you are trying to get or stay lean for racing. Here are some easy and simple light meals (or large snacks) that work well for **longer runs**.

- Medium sweet potato with 2 tablespoons almond butter: 320 calories, 39 grams carbs, 9 grams protein, **ratio of 4.33**
- 1/2 cup (measured dry) oatmeal, 1/4 cup walnuts, 2 tablespoons (about 12) dried tart cherries: 420 calories, 47 grams carbs, 11 grams protein, **ratio 4.2**
- 2 slices whole wheat bread (I like Dave's Killer Bread), 2 tablespoons all-natural peanut butter, and 1 tablespoon all-fruit jelly: 475 calories, 61 grams carbs, 18 grams protein, **ratio 3.38**
- 2 oz (measured dry) whole wheat pasta, 1/4 cup tomato sauce, 1 cup broccoli, 2/3 cup green peas: 381 calories, 68 grams carbs, 15.6 grams protein, **ratio of 4.3**
- 1/4 (measured dry) cup quinoa, 1/2 cup pinto beans, 1 cup broccoli, 2/3 cup green peas: 378 calories, 69.4 grams carbs, 21.3 grams protein, **ratio 3.25**

I could go on forever! If you don't want to be bothered by grams and ratios, the easy shortcut to remember is "nuts with fruit" and "beans and greens." (Broccoli, peas, kale, and other green vegetables have a huge percentage of protein per gram.) It doesn't need to be complicated or exact. In fact, the simpler it is, the better, both for your body and for convenience.

Does that mean that I never use packaged bars? Sometimes I do. But I don't like relying on them, especially when it's just as easy to eat real whole food.

The trick to recovering after gym workouts is to plan ahead so you can easily have several options on hand that taste great, offer carbs and protein, curb the appetite, and keep you from reaching for the junk food or driving through the fast-food window.

Now, I'm not suggesting that you devote every Sunday meal prepping like a maniac, unless that works for you. The simplest option is to simply double your recipes when you cook so that you can freeze your leftovers in single-serve portions. That way you'll always have something homemade and delicious just a few minutes away with hardly any extra work.

But the main thing to remember is that the best recovery foods are not just the ones that you eat immediately after a workout. Eating a plant-rich diet of colorful fruits and vegetables along with nuts, seeds, and whole grains will give your body the fiber and micro-nutrients it needs to stay healthy and grow strong lean muscles. It doesn't mean that you can't have a cookie every once in a while, but the vast majority of what you eat should be whole, unprocessed food, so you can spend less time recovering and more time running!

How to Actually Lose Weight by Running

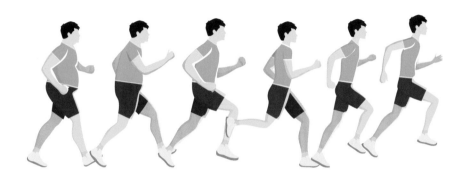

Many people, myself included, picked up the running habit with one goal in mind: to lose weight. While the benefits of running can go far beyond losing a few pounds, running can be a fantastic part of your strategy to get in the best shape of your life.

So why is it that runners come in all shapes and sizes? If running is so good for weight loss, why aren't all runners perfectly trim and lean? And what about those stories that you hear of people actually gaining weight while training for the marathon? (I did!) How is that even possible when you are pounding out mile after mile?

The easy answer is that these runners must just be eating too much food. After all, the only way to lose weight is to burn more calories than you consume. That's just physics.

So the simple solution is to eat less and run more and voila, perfect beach body guaranteed. But so often it just doesn't seem to work that way. So how do you actually lose weight with running?

Beyond Calories In and Calories Out

Let's dive a little deeper beyond just calories in and calories out to explore why you might not be losing weight despite how much you run. Then I'll go over how you can change your routine and habits to finally achieve the results you are looking for.

Our bodies are adaptable, which is great, because that means we can become better at running. But if you are running purely for weight loss, you'll have to keep running more and more and more to get the same calorie burn as you did when you were an awkward and heavier beginner.

As you lose weight from running, you will not need as many calories to move through life, so your energy needs go down, meaning you need to eat even less to continue the weight loss. And it turns out, your body really doesn't like to lose weight quickly, so it turns the fire down on your metabolism even further than your fancy watch or your fitness tracker would like us to believe.

So we run more, even though we are burning fewer calories per mile. If we are not aware that this is happening, we will continue to eat the same way and wonder why our weight has plateaued. But the really tricky thing is that even if we are perfectly aware of this phenomenon, we might still easily overcompensate with extra calories.

Compensation for Exercise

Compensation is the conscious or unconscious intake or absorption of more calories after a session of exercise. That could mean having an extra brownie or two after your long run because you've told yourself you deserve it. Or that could be your body purposely ramping up your hunger hormones, suppressing your fullness hormones, and increasing your desire hormones, making that brownie absolutely irresistible.

While this is undoubtedly frustrating, don't hang up your running shoes just yet. Countless people have lost lots of weight with running. So how do they do it? What makes those runners different from the marathon runners that actually gain weight? I'll get into that part next.

Focus on Your First Priority First

When trying to lose weight with running, you should first yourself what your personal goals are. Is weight loss the main priority and you just happen to like running? Or is running the priority and weight loss would be nice, too? Because the way you approach your running and your weight loss should be very different depending on your answer.

If you want to run faster and farther and happen to have some weight to lose, the best way to do that is to separate the two goals into different periods in the year. Just like weightlifters and football players have bulk phases and cut phases, you will want to plan a time in between specific race training cycles to lose weight.

This ensures you aren't in a calorie deficit when you are trying to build muscle and endurance for performance. For trained athletes, regardless of their weight status, it is incredibly difficult to lose fat and gain muscle at the same time. Not to mention that underfueling is an express train to injury.

When weight loss is your goal, your running, training, and nutrition will look different than when performance is your top priority. Of course, if you are a beginner runner, you can lose weight and get much better at running at the same time, but running should be part of the goal and not the entire goal itself.

Add Walking

As a new runner, you'll want to ease into a running routine. Increase your running frequency, intensity, and distance gradually (and one at a time) to lower the risk of injury and get the best results. Because running is high-impact, overuse injuries are common if you add too much too soon, and unfortunately, the risk of injury is even higher for heavier runners.

A great way to mitigate the risk of injury and still burn lots of calories is to incorporate walking. Compared to running, walking is less stressful on the bones, muscles, and joints, but it's still stressful enough to create beneficial adaptations that will improve your ability to handle more running.

You might start off by walking only or with a mix of walking and running. Once things start to feel a bit easier after a few weeks, gradually shift the balance further and further toward running until you are comfortable with all running. The overall goal should be to aim for 300 minutes of brisk walking or running each week.

Bump Up Your Strength Training

The next key part of weight loss and body recomposition is strength training. Not only will strong muscles help you become a better, more resilient runner, but muscle is more metabolically expensive than fat. That means muscle will require more calories to grow and maintain, helping you burn more calories all day long.

A good strength program will work all of the major muscle groups, and you should aim for about 60 minutes per week of lifting, which should be broken up into two or more sessions per week.

Boost Your Intensity

Another calorie torcher is high intensity interval training, or HIIT. This could be done by incorporating speedier intervals into your run once a week or with a separate plyometric or jumping session per week. HIIT has been shown to promote weight loss and is great for creating power in runners, but because of its intensity level, it should only be done about once a week.

Focus on Nutrition

Now that we have the exercise plan down, we have to talk about your diet. Many people will say that I have it backwards and the food side is more important. Technically, that is probably true, and I'm sure you have heard the phrase "you can't outrun a bad diet." But focusing on deprivation can make success that much harder.

Kate Salina, a writer who lost 65 pounds with running, became a runner first without trying to change her diet. Rather than seeing running as simply a weight-loss tool, Kate chose to see running as something that could play a positive role in all aspects of her life and not just for what it could do on the scale.

"When I began running," she wrote in a 2020 article for *Medium*, "I deliberately focused on the running aspect rather than the weight loss element—and I did not consciously focus on my diet. The problem with trying to fix your diet while also starting to run is that you are asking yourself to do two tasks that both require limited willpower."

In the first couple months of running, she noticed her energy levels rising and her moods becoming much better, which resulted in fewer cravings. She lost 20 pounds over the first two months, which she admits was partly due to water weight, but the success gave her the motivation to keep going and make better food choices moving forward.

Running Is the Reward

For Kate, running became the reward, not the punishment, and that is a mental mind shift every runner can benefit from. We don't reward ourselves with junk food. We treat ourselves well with good running and good whole food.

That means we replace processed food like white flour and oils with more fruits, vegetables, lean proteins, and whole food. Swapping out low-quality food with whole, high-nutrient foods will make you feel fuller, and you'll naturally cut calories when you make the switch.

High-quality foods with all their micronutrients and fiber are less energy dense and more satiating than low-quality, processed foods, so they fill you up with fewer calories. By increasing your overall diet quality, you can eat enough to satisfy your heightened appetite while still creating the calorie deficit required for weight loss.

Once you start training again for performance instead of weight loss, you still want to focus on high-quality whole foods, but you'll want to begin to eat a little more of them.

Weight loss with running has been successful for many people, and it all starts in the mind. Take a good look at your goals, your habits, and how you treat yourself, and you can achieve what you set your mind to.

Why You Might Gain Weight While Marathon Training

It seems absolutely counterintuitive, not to mention wholeheartedly unfair, that you can actually gain weight while training for a marathon. But it can be true for some people, and I'm one of them, so this topic hits home for me. So I'd like to go into why this happens, how to avoid it, and why not all weight gain is a bad thing (strange as that sounds).

Muscle Gain

The first reason the scale might be going up instead of down is if you are gaining muscle. This is particularly common with newer marathoners whose body composition can change quite dramatically with the increase in training. So while a pound of muscle weighs exactly the same as a pound of fat (or a pound of feathers), it looks a whole lot different on your body since muscle is more dense.

Presumably, the muscle you are gaining is muscle that helps propel you down the road farther and faster, so muscle gain is rarely a bad thing. But there is also a reason that elite marathoners don't look like bodybuilders. Too much muscle, especially upper body muscle, doesn't help move your body faster after a certain point, so it can literally weigh you down.

But if you are training properly for a marathon, gaining huge muscle mass is quite challenging to do, unless you are spending the same amount of time weight lifting as you are running while also eating lots of extra calories.

Running is a catabolic exercise, meaning that your body breaks down tissue to do it. When you eat and rest after running, your body builds and repairs. If you keep your calorie intake in balance with what you burn, you will not gain huge muscles or get super skinny, unless that's your natural body type.

Fat Gain

If all marathoners' weight gain was attributed to gaining muscle, we probably wouldn't be having this conversation. While some runners do worry about gaining any kind of weight—muscle or fat or something else—most runners are really only concerned about gaining fat.

Fat is essential for human life, of course, but extra fat makes running harder and presumably makes us slower on the race course, right? So let's get as lean as possible to nail those PRs! First of all, that's not exactly true, but I'll talk about that part in a minute.

Before even getting to the discussion about getting super lean, I first want to talk about how to avoid gaining fat when training, assuming that you are at a healthy weight or perhaps heavier than recommended for your height.

How can you gain fat while running more than ever? Because your metabolism is a tricky, moving target, which favors inertia over change. Your body hates change, both good and bad, and fights to keep you exactly where you were yesterday, with lots of sneaky tools at its disposal.

The reason for fat gain is simple and complex at the same time. It's simple because the only way to gain fat is to eat more than you burn. It's complex because you might not even realize that you are doing it.

When you go out and run 15 miles for the first time ever, it's a big deal. You are proud of yourself, you are tired, and you are hungry. So you celebrate with an entire sheet of brownies and a gallon of margaritas. Okay, maybe you don't do that every time, but rewarding yourself with food or drink after exercise can lead to unexpected fat gains for two reasons: One, you are consuming more than you think you are, and two, you are burning less than you think you are.

As you shift from a less active person to a highly active person, your body fights to remain who you used to be. It's not happy when you start to burn off the precious energy stores that it has frantically built up over the years. So when you fill your belly with sleeves of Double Stuffed Oreos and a half a dozen IPAs, your body greedily squirrels it away in your fat cells along with a little something extra in case you get the silly idea to go running again.

Sneak Up on Your Fitness

The trick is to sneak up on your fitness so your body doesn't notice that you are dramatically changing your life. Build mileage slowly and gradually, run slowly on your easy days, be sure you are recovering, and don't overly reward yourself for a job well done with food.

There is room for treats in a healthy lifestyle, but if you are rewarding yourself every day, that's not a treat, that's a habit. Make whole, fresh food the convenient choice, and don't have junk food in the house.

Okay, so let's say you have that part down and your diet is pretty good. Why else would you gain weight?

Overfueling

Let's take a look at how you are fueling your workouts. Are you having a pre-run snack, then sucking down energy gels during your run, then finishing it with a 32-ounce Gatorade, all for your 30-minute easy run? Oops. Fueling properly is important, and refueling after your run is, too, but so many runners go way overboard here, especially on easy runs. Your body is already carrying enough fuel in your muscles for about 90 minutes of running, so you don't have to think about fueling for short, easy runs. It's important for hard, intense speed days or long, long runs, but if you are barely breaking a sweat, put the gel down, and wait until your next normal meal to eat.

Another reason for weight gain in endurance runners is that well fueled muscles are heavier than depleted ones. As you train more and more, your body learns to store more glycogen in your muscles to fuel your runs. So your muscles actually begin to weigh more. And with every gram of glycogen stored, your body stores two to three grams of water. For runners, this is a very good thing, because you need both glycogen and water on board to run long distances well, but that weight will show up on the scale.

At this point, some of you are saying, "Coach Claire, I'm doing all the right things, eating a whole foods diet, not drinking my calories, and not overfueling, and I'm still gaining weight. What gives?"

If that's the case, there could be a couple of things going on. If you've recently lost a good bit of weight and now are gaining or plateauing, what might be happening is that you are now burning fewer calories at rest due to your smaller size. If you lost the weight quickly, your body is now on high alert and is storing and absorbing more calories than it used to when food was abundant.

That means, if you want to break the plateau, you either need to eat less or burn more, both of which are challenging to do when you need to be properly fueled to run well. Run too much, and you risk injury and overtraining. Eat too little, and you are more tired and will underperform.

This is when you need to prioritize your goals. Is your main goal to lose weight? Or are you trying to lose weight so that you can race better? If losing weight is more important than performance, then cutting a few calories without being overly restrictive is the way to go so that you lose it slowly and your body doesn't have time to freak out.

Good Training Is Far More Important Than Weight Loss

If you are at a healthy weight, and you are trying to lose a couple of pounds to shave a few seconds off your marathon time, you are focusing on the wrong metric. Training and experience will make you a far better marathoner than simply having as little body fat as possible.

I know this from personal experience because I fell into the trap of trying to be as tiny as possible to run my fastest. So I tracked every calorie I ate for months to get down to what I thought was my magic race weight of 108 pounds. It worked, and I beat my personal record (PR). Naturally, I thought I was so smart and disciplined, so I tried it again for the next race. But the same techniques no longer worked, and my body was having none of that nonsense. I found myself needing to cut even more calories to get the same results, and it still didn't work. I simply could not get that skinny again without starving myself, and I knew enough to realize that eating 1000 calories a day while training was a stupid thing to do. So for my next race, I was a little heavier, but I had great training and more experience. And I PRd again.

So then I thought, okay, now 113 is my race weight, so I need to get down to that weight again. And surprise, surprise, nothing I did worked. Again, I raced heavier and still performed better.

This pattern of train and gain continued for me until my last marathon, where I finally achieved my dream goal time weighing in at nearly the exact same weight as I did before I even started running. Granted, my body composition was night and day better than before I started running, but my point is that your weight, that number on the scale, is not the point. Being fit and strong will make you far faster than being skinny and weak.

Not to mention that you will be a far nicer person to be around when you are actually eating enough food. Being as lean as possible is a huge commitment that will affect your relationships, how you celebrate, and how you spend your time, so really think about how important those last couple of pounds are to you.

I promise you that you can be fit and fast without starvation or obsessively worrying about the scale. Keep it simple by focusing on whole foods and mostly or entirely plants, and keep the easy days easy and the hard days hard.

Chapter Four

Hydration in All Seasons

We tend to think a lot more about what to drink and how much to drink when it's hot and sunny out. But the truth is that we need to be aware of our hydration needs all year round to get the most out of our running and our performance.

Drink to Thirst (Mostly)

The big question for most runners on this subject is, "How much should I drink?" The simplest and perhaps most effective answer to that is drink when you are thirsty. Your body's sense of thirst is a very important key to your survival as an individual and of our species in general, so it has evolved over the millennia to do a pretty great job at telling you that it's time to drink.

So, if you take away nothing else from this chapter, "drink to thirst" is almost always the best advice.

Notice I said "almost." The advice to drink when you are thirsty might be great if every time you ran, you had a support crew riding next to you on a bike handing you a customized water bottle every time the urge to drink came to mind. For most of us, that's just not reality, and we need to plan our hydration in advance. So we need to know how much we need on a given run.

There are quite a few factors that go into figuring out this puzzle, including how hot it is, how humid it is, how hard you are running, how long you are running, how big you are, how much you sweat, what you ate for breakfast, your overall diet, how heat-adapted you are, your fitness level, your age, your gender, and probably 10 other variables that I haven't even thought of yet.

I won't be getting into every single one of these topics, but don't worry, we'll still be able to come up with a hydration plan that fits you on every run.

Hydration Is Highly Individual

First, let's look inside your body and see what is going on with your fluid levels and why this is important.

Your body is about 80 percent water, so clearly, proper water balance is key to just about every human function. Your body takes in water not only through the liquids you drink but also from the liquid-rich foods that you eat, most notably fruits and vegetables.

When the water comes in through food and drink, it either gets used right away or it gets stored. With each gram of carbohydrate you eat, your body will store two, three, or even four grams of water along with it.

This is good because when you are running and burning glycogen for fuel, you will be freeing up the stored water at the same time, which enables you to maintain the proper fluid balance in your body despite the fact you are sweating buckets.

That means that even if you go on a run and lose two, three, or four pounds of water weight through sweating, you might not actually be dehydrated at all. Sounds a little crazy, but it could be true. Except when it's not! There are other runners that will lose a pound or two and be desperately thirsty and dehydrated. What's going on?

Well, the scientific answer is that we don't really know. Some people seem to be more sensitive to fluid loss than others, and it's not clear why. Many people seem to lose sensitivity to thirst as they age, but that's not true across the board. Other people who have either intentionally or accidentally trained themselves to run with less water eventually become used to drinking less and might not feel as thirsty.

So how do we figure this out for ourselves, and is it even really that important?

Research has shown that during exercise lasting one hour or less, dehydration does not decrease endurance performance, so that means you can skip the water stations when running a 5k at any pace. If your race or run is longer than an hour, drinking according to thirst maximizes endurance performance.

However, the mind plays a big role in this equation. Let's say you are running a marathon and you suddenly feel thirsty and you just passed the water stop without stopping. Simply being under stress worrying about your fluid intake can detract from your performance, so drinking according to a plan can help.

Unfortunately, some runners have been consumed with fear about dehydration. Ignoring their bodies' signals and only drinking to a plan no matter what can lead to a fatal condition called hyponatremia.

So what's the plan to avoid drinking too much but also avoid dehydration? Well, the best advice is to go for a run longer than an hour and find out! Run with a hydration vest or belt or along a route that has plenty of water fountains. Or run on a track with a water bottle at the start line and note when you get thirsty.

The only problem with that is there are so many variables with weather and time of day and speed that it takes a lot of trial and error to get it just right.

The calculations will involve weighing yourself before and after a run and taking into account the fluid you drank during the run as well as any urine loss (have fun measuring that one!), how many calories you burn per mile (and it's not 100 calories per mile for everyone), what your carbohydrate intake is, and more.

And then you will have to do that at every temperature, because you clearly will lose less fluid through sweat in 40 degrees versus 90. It's exhausting just thinking about it!

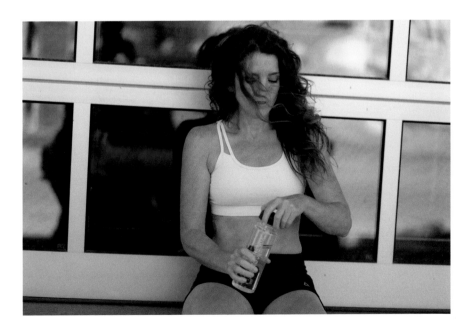

So let's say you don't want or have time to go through all those calculations. How do you know how much to drink during your runs and races?

The unsatisfying answer is trial and error.

No calculator, estimator, or internet blog can tell you exactly how many ounces of liquid you personally will need to avoid detrimental dehydration in a race. Being an experiment of one and noting how you feel at different intake levels is truly the best way to find a hydration plan that works best for you.

There are, however, some important hydration guidelines that can help craft the right plan for you, especially in the summer.

The Best Hydration Plan for Hot Running and Racing

Ah, summer. The warm, sunny days and short nights are perfect for getting outside and savoring nature with family and friends. But if you are an endurance runner, you'll need a hydration plan for hot running and racing.

Not only is running simply more uncomfortable as the mercury rises, but the combination of heat, sun, humidity, and distance will begin to affect our performance as the body struggles to cool itself down.

If you've ever come back from a run soaked in sweat, or had salt stinging your eyes and staining your clothes, you probably already know that hydration is important. And if you are training this summer for a marathon or an ultra, a solid hydration plan is an absolute must.

Runs and Races Under 60 Minutes

If your runs, workouts, or races are less than an hour, even if you are sweating puddles, coming up with a perfect hydration protocol is not super important to health and performance. You do not need to replenish with gallons of Gatorade after a short jog or a sweaty strength session. Simply drinking to thirst when you are done with the run is usually sufficient to bring your fluid levels back to normal.

And it's easy to recharge your electrolyte balance with healthy whole foods after your workout, no special drinks or solutions required. If you notice that you are a very salty sweater, enjoying some lightly salted foods after a run will probably do the trick.

But once you get into runs and workouts that go longer than an hour, or if you are training for a multi-hour event, it's time to get a more focused hydration strategy for maximum performance.

Runs and Races Longer Than an Hour

Besides being thirsty and uncomfortable, dehydration will start to affect your performance. Water (along with sodium) is what keeps your blood flowing quickly and easily to your heart, lungs, and muscles. Not to mention that it's essential for every cell in the body to function.

When you become dehydrated, your blood becomes thicker, which makes your heart work harder, which, in turn, makes running harder. If you offset your sweat loss by drinking on the run, you can race further and faster without slowing down.

But how do we know exactly how much to drink? And exactly what? Theories on hydration for endurance have oscillated wildly over the years, and most experts tell us to begin with our thirst.

Drink to Thirst (Sort Of)

Our thirst mechanism is highly attuned to making sure that we maintain homeostasis, or a perfect balance of fluid to electrolytes. When we sweat, we eventually get thirsty and might even crave salt as our body's signal to eat and drink.

But during a long endurance event, our thirst might not be quite as reliable the longer the race goes on. We are less able to absorb calories and liquids as the blood gets diverted to the skin and away from the gut. So we need to start fueling and hydrating BEFORE we are thirsty.

During most marathons, aid stations are easy to come by, and you can plan to drink every two to three miles or so, more often if it's hot. With longer ultras or less-supported races, you'll want to plan to carry what you need between aid stations.

Either way, a plan is essential.

Plan for Success

The first step is finding out how much you sweat. Most runners already know if they are on the sweatier end of the spectrum, but it's also a good idea to get some better data on just how much sweat is lost.

Getting a rough idea of your sweat rate is pretty simple. You just weigh yourself naked before a hot run, weigh yourself when you get back, and subtract any liquid you drank on the run. The result is your sweat loss on a similar run. This is not lab-precise because you lost more than just water on the run, but it's close enough to determine if you are a heavy sweater or not.

Next, you'll need to figure out how much you need to replace while running. This will be quite subjective because the costs of dehydration are different for everyone. Some runners will get slowed down by as little as a one percent loss of body weight, while other runners can handle up to an eight percent sweat loss.

In general, most people do not start to see performance declines until about three to four percent.

Now that does not mean that you want to replace 100 percent of the fluid you lost. That would lead to a sloshing belly and would probably decrease your ability to run well. So you'll have to keep experimenting on your runs to find the right amount of liquid you can comfortably handle.

Pre-Hydration

One overlooked part of your hydration plan is to start off fully hydrated. It can make a big difference in how quickly you dehydrate. It is similar to the concept of carb-loading, but because the body cannot store water in the same way it stores fuel, it's done a little differently.

The downside of pre-hydrating and carb-loading? Weight gain.

Most runners hate to learn that they should aim to start a race weighed down with water and glycogen. As a coach, I hear from a lot of runners that are worried about how the extra weight will slow them down. But the truth is exactly the opposite. With fully topped off stores of fuel and hydration, you have what you need exactly where you need it, giving you a performance edge.

Sodium Is Key

Sodium intake is critical to any hydration plan, but that can be a tough concept to fully embrace, especially among healthy runners that have chosen to follow a healthy lifestyle with naturally low-sodium foods. But unless your doctor has told you to limit your sodium intake (and you've told your doctor how much you run), you might want to reconsider the role sodium plays in your running and your diet.

Much like how simple sugars are a bad idea for a sedentary adult but the perfect fuel for racing, sodium's impact on dehydration cannot be understated. A typical runner can lose anywhere from 250 to over 1000 milligrams of sodium per liter of sweat. If you sweat two liters of sweat per hour and are a salty sweater, you've lost almost all of your sodium requirement for the entire day (the RDA is 2300 milligrams)!

That does not give runners a free pass to eat as much sodium as they like, however. But you do need to be aware of its importance to your overall hydration plan for endurance.

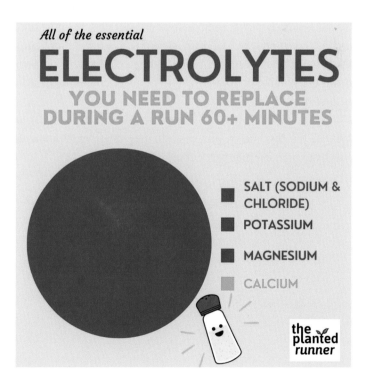

While figuring out your sweat rate is pretty straightforward, figuring out your exact sodium loss rate is not quite as simple without a lab test. But research has found that a very subjective self-survey ends up being fairly accurate. In other words, if your running clothes have white salt streaks on them or your sweat stings your eyes when you run, you most likely do have a higher-than-average sodium loss.

The Rest of the Electrolytes

With all this talk about sodium, you might be wondering, what about the rest of the electrolytes? Pick up a bottle of any sports drink designed for endurance and you will see a list of other minerals like potassium, magnesium, and calcium, which are all essential electrolytes.

Despite what the bottle says, you don't need any of those while running, unless perhaps you are running a multi-day stage race. Sodium is king because it's the only one that is lost in significant quantities in sweat. The rest can be consumed with real food when you are done running.

Test and Tweak

The last step in your perfect hydration plan is to test and experiment as often as you can. Try out a slightly higher sodium drink on your next hot long run and note how it goes. Test it out on a fast workout, even if it is less than an hour long, and see if it makes any difference. Adjust, tweak, and record the results in your training log throughout the summer until you find the combination of fluid to sodium levels that suits you best.

By the time you toe the line of your marathon or ultra, you'll know your exact hydration needs to produce your best performance. No sweat.

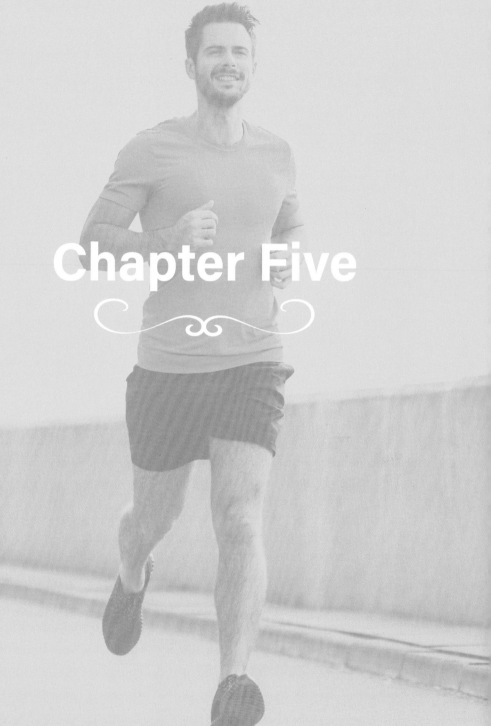

Chapter Five

Build on Your Skills

How to introduce speed, lengthen your runs, and stay injury free

How to Run Faster

Just about every runner, whether you run 5-minute miles or 12-minute miles, wants to become faster. Running fast is fun, and the sense of accomplishment you get when you run faster than ever is absolutely thrilling. So how do you actually do it? Well, there are lots of ways that you can get better and faster at running, no matter where you start. Obviously, in order to run faster, you need to run fast. In other words, you need to do some speed work. But speed work is only part of the puzzle, so let's talk about the rest of the pieces.

Run More (But Not Too Much)

Like just about anything in life, the more you do something, the better you get at it. But unfortunately, you can't just keep adding miles into infinity. There will be a point where running more is detrimental to your progress, not to mention the rest of your life, so the key here is to add mileage in a smart, gradual way.

If you currently run three times a week, try adding in an additional day with a short, easy run. A rule of thumb that gets tossed around is to not increase your mileage more than 10 percent a week, and for most people, that's probably pretty safe, but that calculation can get a bit skewed at the higher levels.

Adding to the frequency of your runs is probably the single most effective way to increase your running fitness level because it stimulates your metabolism more regularly, and it's less taxing to run shorter more often rather than longer less frequently.

If you are happy with the frequency of your runs, it's time to add a little length to your runs. Depending on what type of race you are training for, you might add a little to an easy mid-week run, or you might add to your long run. Again, the key here is to add mileage so gradually that the body doesn't realize what you are doing. The best way to build fitness is to sneak up on it!

Run Slower on Easy Days

The second way to run faster is not so obvious. In fact, it's completely counterintuitive. If you want to run fast, you also need to learn how to run SLOW. As I mentioned in the previous chapter, the vast majority of recreational runners run their easy days way too fast. What that does is keeps you in the mid-range of your ability all the time. Your runs are not fast enough to stimulate growth or improvement, yet they are too fast to get the recovery benefits. Most people actually end up needing recovery days to recover from their recovery days!

Running very easy on easy days allows you to build mileage safely so you can run more with less down time.

How slow is slow? As I mentioned earlier, your easy day should be, at a bare minimum, at least one minute slower than your marathon pace and preferably slower than that. My easy runs are typically two minutes slower than my marathon pace, and many days are even slower. But the key here is not to focus on pace on easy days. Save that for your hard workout days. You need to focus on a slow and easy effort.

If you can breathe entirely out of your nose the whole run or sing along out loud to your music or chat with your running buddy as easily as you could walking, you are going slow enough, no matter what your watch says.

And if that means you have to stop and catch your breath or even walk for a few minutes, that's exactly what you need to do. There's no ego on easy days.

So while you are logging all these easy miles, what's going on to make you faster? Well, besides gaining fitness, your body is figuring out how to get you down the road in the most efficient way possible. Yes, there are some well-researched ways to improve your form to increase efficiency, but the body hates inefficiency and will figure out a way to run in such a way that burns the least amount of energy without you having to think about it.

That being said, a more efficient runner is a faster runner in endurance running (the opposite is actually true for sprinters), so consciously working on your form during easy runs helps. Use a light, quick cadence no matter your pace, and keep your torso tall and relaxed with your shoulders down, head looking forward, and arms close to the body and moving forward rather than side to side.

Strong Runners Are Faster Runners

The next piece of the puzzle is strength training (more in chapter six). I consider strength training vital to not only becoming a faster runner but to becoming less injury prone and more durable. That means that since your legs are a bit tougher when you go out for a run, you are not as sore afterwards, and you might not need as much recovery, meaning you can run again sooner without pain. It doesn't take much. You can do 10 minutes a day or two good sessions a week.

Another tip is to add in some hill work (more on this later in the chapter). Running up and down hills is strength and speed work in disguise, even at a slow pace. The added resistance you have fighting gravity on the uphill builds strong leg muscles, and the eccentric muscle contractions on the downhill increases leg durability and has been proven to decrease delayed onset muscle soreness. If you want to up the ante on hills, you can try some hill repeats, which is where you run hard up a hill for 30 seconds or so and walk back down for recovery.

Nutrition and Body Composition

Next, you must take a look at your nutrition and body weight. If your diet is full of healthy, whole, unprocessed foods, then it's highly likely that you are able to maintain a healthy body weight and can properly fuel your life and your training to become fit and fast. If you are overweight, running is much harder, and you will be slower. Science is showing us that exercise alone is a poor method for losing weight, so make sure that your food is truly nourishing and you don't routinely overdo it.

That being said, losing too much weight will end up slowing you down as well. Undernourished athletes suffer from fatigue and lack of motivation and are at a higher risk of injury, so be sure not to cross the line into underfueling. Proper training and nutrition will beat out low body weight and underfueling every time.

Cross Training

My next tip for you is another seemingly counterintuitive one: Maybe you actually need to run less to get faster. Some people, especially as they age, simply can't handle the pounding of running day after day. More is not better at some point.

But that doesn't mean you should be lying on the couch more; it means you should be cross training. That could be as simple as going for a walk with your dog, swimming some easy laps, or going to a spin class. Aerobic cross training helps build up your aerobic engine while giving your bones and tendons a break from the high-impact forces of running.

Another sneaky way cross training helps is that it builds up your non-running muscles so they can then serve as additional storage centers for the glycogen needed to run long distances. It's like getting another gas tank!

Run With Friends

My last suggestion is to find your tribe. Running with a buddy or with a training group is incredibly motivating and inspiring. It's the good kind of peer pressure that can keep you training during the dark days of winter and the hot days of summer. Most towns have group runs or track workouts that you can join that are open to all paces and abilities, so there's bound to be one filled with people just like you.

Adding in a Sprinkle of Speed

While lots of easy running is the most important part of becoming better at endurance running, to truly reach your potential, you will have to run faster at times. Most experts recommend that 80 percent of your running should be at an easy pace, while 20 percent of your runs can be speed days.

But that doesn't mean that you should just run all-out until you fall to the ground once a week. Specific workouts at certain speeds can predictably develop your fitness level with far less risk of injury.

Strides

What if I told you that there was a way to get faster, improve your running form, quicken your feet, better prepare for a race, *and* have some fun, all with less than 90 seconds of work? I'd say sign me up.

The good news is that such a thing actually exists. This simple speed development drill is a staple of track and field and cross-country teams all over the world and can massively improve running, yet many recreational runners are missing out it. It's called the *stride*. Or striders, or accelerations, or stride-outs. Lots of names for the same awesome skill. But what it's not is a sprint or a surge. I'll get to those a little bit later.

If you are a beginner, they are the absolute best way to begin with speed. If you've been running a while but have never tried strides, they can help break you out of a plateau. And if you are a masters runner, strides are simply the best way to maintain and perhaps even improve your skills and speed as you age.

Running strides benefits every runner at every stage. Even if you've been doing strides for years, this is a perfect refresher to reinforce everything you've been doing right for your running! And you just might learn a new tip to perfect them.

What Are Strides?

Strides are 20 to 35 seconds of very fast running. It is not an all-out, chased-by-a-tiger effort, but rather 85 to 90 percent of all-out effort. If you want to attach a race-pace effort, it's about your mile race pace, but I always hesitate to use race paces to describe the pace of a particular drill like strides.

The reason for that is primarily because most people have no idea what their one-mile race pace is. Even if you decided to go find out how fast you could run a mile by heading out to your local high school track tomorrow, that's not going to be accurate. Why? Because unless you've spent weeks or months or even years specifically training for the mile, whatever you run alone on the track is not representative of your potential at the mile.

But even if you know precisely what your best mile race pace is down to the tenth of a second, it makes zero difference when it comes to your stride pace. And that's because strides are not about pace. They are not even about speed.

It's better to think of them as a speed development drill. You are practicing running fast so you can get better at running fast. How fast you actually run a stride is not the point. How well you run a stride is.

But before I get to exactly how you do your strides right, let's talk about why you should incorporate them into your running in the first place.

Why You Should Run Strides

Strides have a ton of benefits, and there are five main reasons to use them.

1. Strides help you work on running mechanics and excellent form in short little pieces. It's hard to stay 100 percent present and focused on running your best all the time. But with 20- or 30-second strides, you can micromanage all the little form details with your full attention. Since strides are done after an easy run or before a hard workout, your body and your brain aren't too tired to pay attention with laser focus.
2. Strides are the perfect introduction to speed for beginner runners. If you are just starting out, the thought of running a mile or two at any pace is challenging, let alone trying an intimidating speed session that you are simply not ready for. Strides are a perfect way to get to know what fast running feels like, and they can jump start your progression into speedier workouts.
3. Strides add a little spicy speed to the legs of long-distance runners. Because most of your runs either need to be slow to build up your aerobic system or at tempo pace to build stamina, marathoners' legs can feel a bit stale after weeks of training. Strides offer you a great way to inject some speed work into your training plan without having to sacrifice a whole day of training. Just a few strides a couple of days a week can sprinkle in some fast footwork without sacrificing specific training.
4. Strides are a perfect drill to add into your warm-up routine for your speed days and races. After 10 to 20 minutes of jogging, add some strides and other form drills before you start your intervals or your race. The burst of speed will remind the legs there is work to do and get the adrenaline pumping.
5. And finally, strides are FUN! There's nothing like flying down the road pretending you are Usain Bolt or Allyson Felix. Running fast is fun, and strides make you feel fast. (If only for a few seconds.)

As you practice strides over weeks and months, you no longer have to concentrate quite so hard, because great form while running fast is starting to feel more normal. And that will eventually translate to more natural fast running on race day.

What is the best way to do strides? Remember, I said they are not a sprint and not a surge. So what the heck are they?

The Three Phases of a Stride

A common misconception about strides is that they are sprints. Let's imagine elite sprinters racing the 100-meter dash. They start at zero and explode as fast as possible, reaching their peak speed as they cross the finish line and only slowing down when the race is over.

Strides are different. They are not sprints. A better image to keep in your head is a bell curve.

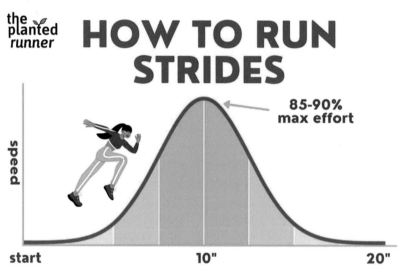

the planted runner

HOW TO RUN STRIDES

85-90% max effort

speed

start   10"   20"

Strides are a surprisingly powerful way to improve your running without needing a recovery day!

Add four 20 second strides after an easy run or use them as a drill before a hard workout or race.

Start by running hard with great form. Reach near-max speed halfway, then ease back down.

Stop after each one and let your breathing come back down to normal (2-3 minutes) before starting your next stride.

The First Five Seconds

For your 20 second stride, you begin accelerating into your fast pace over the first 5 seconds. It is important to ease into the pace and not explode into top speed to prevent injury. After 5 seconds, you should have reached full speed. This is where you will try to stay for the middle of the stride, or about 10 seconds.

The Middle 10 Seconds

During this 10-second window of fast (but not all out) running, your goal is to stay 100 percent present and focused on the important work you are doing. This is where you are practicing your very best running, and it is far more effective if you are paying attention.

In these 10 seconds, your body will do its best to find the most efficient way to run fast for you. That will look slightly different for every runner, but there are some universal form cues that you can keep in mind to help this process along.

Focus on staying relaxed and letting your body do the work. Avoid the natural temptation to grimace or grind your teeth when you are working hard. This wastes unnecessary energy in your face and will be a harder habit to break later if you unconsciously practice this in training.

A better habit is to keep your face relaxed or even to smile. Smiling while working hard is a scientifically proven painkiller, and strides are a great place to practice this technique.

During the stride, make sure your arms are moving smoothly in a forwards and backwards motion. Your elbows drive high behind your shoulders. Any side to side or cross-body movement with your arms is a missed opportunity to propel you forward.

Instead of clenching your hands into fists, imagine they are blades of steel slicing through the air.

Your entire body should have a noticeable lean forward beginning at the ankles all the way up to your nose. The nose should be the first part of your body to cross an imaginary line. Your big toe should cross last. Your spine is tall and straight, supported by a tight core, and your shoulders are down and back. Consciously think about landing on your midfoot, not your heel, with your knees driving you forward.

Yes, that's a lot to think about in 10 seconds! But the more you do this practice, the more habitual all this positive reinforcement will be.

But even more important than all of these form cues I just gave you is that you stay relaxed. I know for some people the words "relax" and "fast" don't go together, but they actually can. In fact, when you reach the level of fitness where you can run fast and stay relaxed, there is no limit to the possibilities.

The Finish

Continue to stay relaxed at your top end speed. Over the last five seconds, gradually slow yourself to a stop. Take the next couple of minutes to relax and catch your breath and do it again.

What to Do During the Rest

Typically, a set of strides will include four to six strides, with two to three minutes of full rest in between. When you come to the end of your stride, stop completely, catch your breath, and let your heart rate come back down to near normal. Some people stand, others walk, and others prefer to jog slowly back to the starting point.

All of those choices are fine, but if I had to choose, I prefer my athletes not to jog in between. The goal of the rest is full recovery, and that will happen better without the jog. With a full recovery, it's always easier to run faster in any distance, and strides are no exception. So set yourself up for success on each rep and get as recovered as possible.

Strides Are Not the Same as Surges

One common misconception about strides is that they are the same as surges. While they are similar, they are not quite the same thing and do not work on the same skill.

Surges are injections of speed within a run (see chapter nine). When pressed for time, some runners will throw a few surges into the last mile of their easy run and say that they've done their strides. They have not.

A surge practices the skill of running faster when you are tired. It can also be used by competitive runners when trying to shake off rivals in a race. Or it can be used to break up the monotony of a long, flat marathon. These are all good reasons to practice surges, but they are not strides.

Strides, on the other hand, are a speed mechanics tool. You practice running fast in small doses so you get used to running faster in big chunks later. Your body learns its own unique way to be smooth and efficient, and soon, fast running becomes second nature.

Interval Training

Interval training is a type of training in which you alternate short periods of high-intensity effort with less-intense recovery periods. In other words, you break up bits of hard, fast running with slow running. This allows you to spend more time running at high speed because you get enough time to recover so you can do it again.

Obviously, you can run 1 lap around a track at a much faster pace than you could run 4 or 5 or 10 laps around the track, but when you add some jogging or walking breaks, you can run a much longer distance at high speed that you could all at once.

That means your body learns to run at a faster pace and, over time, means that you'll run faster overall. Studies[29] have shown that much greater training effects can be achieved with interval running than with moderate- or medium-intensity running, but a little goes a long way.

Intense intervals improve your aerobic and anaerobic endurance, increase your VO2 max, and improve your running performance.

And, because interval training is such a high stimulus for your muscles, it will take a lot of energy to repair and build muscle tissue after you stop running and start to recover. This effect, where you are burning additional calories as you rest and recover, is known as the afterburn, and can be very helpful if you are trying to lose weight.

So what can possibly go wrong with intervals? Well, the biggest issues with intervals are also the biggest variables in your training overall. And those are intensity, distance, and frequency. In other words, many runners (especially those that are new and excited) run intervals too hard, too long, or too often.

If you are just starting out with intervals and you've never raced before, it can be pretty daunting to attempt a workout that directs you to run 10x400 meter repeats at your 5k pace. What in the world does that mean?

Typically, what a new runner thinks that means is, "race as hard as possible around the track and try not to die by the third one"

There is a better way, however.

Intervals Are Not Sprinting

Keeping your intervals aerobic is best for beginner runners to help build up some general endurance. Try starting out with running hard for just 30 seconds, and then jog for twice as long. And by "running hard while keeping it aerobic," I don't mean run like a tiger is chasing you. Choose a pace for your intervals that you can maintain so you can still run the last interval at the same speed as the first one. In other words, don't sprint. This will take some trial and error at first, but with a little practice, you will learn what this feels like.

When you are done, you should feel like you could do another couple of intervals at the same pace without dying. But it should be hard enough that you really wouldn't want to do much more.

At the beginning, once a week is enough to get you accustomed to interval training. As you become a more experienced runner, you might be able to add a second day a week if you are recovering well in between sessions and feel like your fitness needs the extra stimulation.

Even Splits Are Better Than Fast Splits

A "split" is the time it took you to run one interval. So once you start doing intervals regularly, how do you get even splits? And why are even splits important anyway?

The reason we want to see even splits is because it shows control. Speed is great, but if you can't control it, you can't race well, and you'll end up in a heaping, sweaty mess on the side of the road. Developing patience and control of your speed will teach you how to master it.

Six Tips for Successful Speed Sessions

1. **Realize that everything will get harder as the effort goes on, so purposely sandbag the first few intervals.** In other words, your first intervals should not feel very hard because your last few definitely will at the same pace. Just like any race longer than 800 meters, if you go out too fast, you will pay for it in

the end. It is far better to choose to go slow at the beginning than be forced to slow down at the end.

2. **The middle intervals are often the most mentally challenging.** This is what I like to call the tunnel effect. You are just as far in as you are out, and things are getting real. You have started to tire at this point, and you still have a long way to go. Knowing that most people tend to fade in the middle splits can be just enough motivation to keep your nose to the grindstone.

3. **Wear a watch and use it, but know its limitations.** So many of the newer runners I coach are either entirely dependent on their brand-new GPS watches or have heard about how much better it is to run by feel and don't look at their watches at all. Both types then wonder why their splits are all over the map. First of all, GPS has a terrible time being accurate at the track and has issues with short distances. The best way to time your intervals is to run a measured distance using your watch as a simple timer. A track is best, of course, but any flat route that you know the distance of works great, too.

Learn how to use your lap button (typically the back button on Garmin watches), and click it before and after each interval. Since you are going to use the time elapsed instead of GPS pace, you'll need to figure out what you need to hit in time rather than pace. For example, if you are trying to run your 400s in 8:00 per mile pace, that works out to be just under two minutes per lap.

For a 400, I like to check my watch at the 100-meter mark, then halfway at the 200-meter mark, then click the lap button as I cross the lap line. That way, I can see right away if I'm on pace and can also see if I need to speed up or slow down for the second half.

Another way to look at it is that each interval is just like the whole session in miniature. The first 100 should feel relatively easy, the effort builds in the middle, and the last 100 is high effort, but the end is in sight.

As you get better at this, you might not need to glance at your watch so much, and that's great, but don't be afraid to use it as the tool that it is.

4. **As you run each interval, notice all the little details.** Feel the wind on your face. Notice your breathing patterns. Feel how high your heel comes up behind you. Think about how you are moving your arms to reach a certain speed. Everyone runs a little differently, and learning what your body does at different speeds will teach you what your pace is if you practice it often enough.

5. **Find a rhythm.** As you learn to notice your breathing patterns, you can also begin to find your rhythm at different paces. Some people actually count in their head their steps or their breathing patterns or both.

   If you learn the rhythm of your stride, each step will have the same length and frequency as the last. This is how experienced runners hit their splits on the nose over and over again. Again, it's only possible to do this if your pace is such that your effort feels relatively easy from the beginning. If you are dying after the first interval, you will not be able to hold that intensity the entire workout, so be sure to allow the effort to build up.

6. **Find a group.** If you can, find a group in your town that runs track once a week. This is the absolute best way to learn. Many towns attract runners of all speeds, ages, and abilities, so you are likely to find someone that will be at your level.

TIPS FOR SUCCESSFUL SPEED SESSIONS

1. Sandbag the first few intervals
2. Use your watch, but know its limitations
3. Notice all the details of how it feels
4. The middle intervals can be the toughest
5. Find a rhythm
6. Run with a group or a friend
7. Do your best without stress!

the planted runner

Running with other people also lowers the perception of effort, so you can run harder with less effort. But be warned that just because it felt easier, it wasn't, so be sure to get the recovery you need.

And my last piece of advice on speed days is to just do your best. All running makes you a better runner. If you miss your splits, fade at the end, need a water break in the middle, or have to stop early to get to work, it's all okay. You're still out there getting some good work in, and you will be better because of it.

How to Nail Your Running Paces Just by Feel

Can you tell what pace you are running by feel alone? Most runners have a hard time doing this, but I'll give you a few tips so that you can learn to nail your running paces by feel.

The "Feel" Comes From the Purpose

If you are just starting your running journey, you are probably at the point where you are diving deep into everything running. I know because I've been there!

You might be learning all about tempo runs, steady runs, threshold runs, VO2 max workouts, and more. Maybe you've even joined a group that runs workouts at the local track. Good for you, and welcome to the running community! It's awesome here.

Or maybe you have been running for a while and are starting to feel like a slave to your watch. You don't have a clear sense of what your runs should feel like, other than that you should run fast on speed days.

So let's figure this out.

Let's say that you find a workout that you want to try and it says, "Run half marathon pace for three miles or half marathon effort." That's super helpful if you have just raced a half, but if you've never raced one before, what on earth does that feel like? Or what if you find a workout that simply says, "Run medium effort." Uh, that's not very helpful at all, right?

Let me break this all down a little bit.

The first step is understanding the purpose of each run. That's the key to determining how you should feel for each one. Like anything, learning paces by feel will take time. But you'll get a lot better at it faster if you can understand the "why" of your workout before you even lace up your shoes.

Let's look at some typical runs for distance runners, their purpose, and how you should feel when running them.

Steady State

Steady runs are used for several different purposes, but my favorite use for them is in marathon training. Use steady runs the day before some of your long runs to "pre-fatigue" your legs a little. This will make your long run feel harder without having to run as many miles in one day.

Typically, a steady run is right around marathon pace, but again, if you've never raced a marathon before, that's not helping you much! But I'll get to that part in a second. We have to understand the purpose of the steady before we get too attached to what pace you should run.

Running at your steady pace maximizes development of your aerobic threshold, which is defined as the fastest pace you can run while still remaining completely aerobic. That means your muscles have enough oxygen to produce all the energy they need. At the same time, you are still burning fat as your primary fuel source.

If you go faster than that, you cross the threshold and start to go anaerobic. That can be useful for other workouts, but not the steady state.

Why should you try to stay in the aerobic zone? If you want to run anything longer than a 5k, that will be your primary energy system. More than 85 percent of the energy needed for distances of 5k or longer comes from your aerobic system, so you'll want to get good at it. The more you can develop your aerobic system over months and years of training, the faster you'll be able to run over long distances.

What Does a Steady Feel Like?

The best way to describe it is "comfortably hard." You should be able to run a good chunk of your workout at that pace, but it's not exactly easy. It's around marathon pace, so that might be a pace you could run for three, four, or even five hours. But if you are just starting out, I hope you are not out there running for three to five hours at a time just yet!

But maybe your normal run is, let's say 30 minutes. I'll give you 10 minutes each for the warm-up and cool-down, so that only leaves you 10 minutes. When you are just starting out, your steady pace might be what you can do for those 10 middle minutes. But if you are already fit or have a big aerobic engine from other sports, you might be able to run much faster than what I would call a steady pace, so watch out for that.

"Comfortably hard" is going to mean something different to every runner, so one trick is to use your breathing as a guide to how it should feel.

Steady runs should typically be performed while breathing at a 3:3 ratio (three steps—left, right, left—while breathing in, and three steps while breathing out). A 3:3 breathing rhythm enables you to take about 30 breaths per minute, which is needed for running "comfortably hard."

Another easy way to test whether you're running somewhere in the range of steady pace is to try to talk out loud. If you can get out maybe three to four sentences, but can't talk the ear off your running buddy, that's probably about right. If you can only blurt out one or two sentences before you start gasping for breath, you're running too hard.

Tempo or Lactate Threshold

The tempo run is a classic stamina-building workout for distance runners. I define stamina as speed plus endurance. Running the wrong pace on a tempo, both too slow or too fast, is not going to give you the most bang for your stamina-boosting buck.

Typically, a tempo run is going to come in somewhere around 10-mile race pace and half marathon pace. But that will depend on the distance of the workout, because the longer the run, the harder that pace will be to sustain.

What is the purpose of a tempo? It can help if we call a tempo by its other name, lactate threshold run. That's defined as the fastest pace you can run without generating more lactic acid than your body can utilize and reconvert back into energy.

Your body can only reconvert a certain amount of lactic acid back into energy before it floods the system and contributes to fatigue. That's the burning feeling you get in your legs when you run hard.

If you want to learn to race faster, you must teach your body to clear lactate more efficiently. That's done with this kind of run. But if you run the wrong speed for a tempo, you'll either produce too much lactate quickly (by running too fast) or you'll not produce enough lactate (by running too slow) and not challenge your body.

That is why it's critical that you learn how to feel what tempo pace should be and not just rely on your watch.

What Does a Tempo Feel Like?

A tempo run should feel like a "hard but controlled effort." You should be able to continue your tempo pace for somewhere around 30 to 45 minutes.

The breathing rhythm for a tempo pace is typically a 2:2 ratio (two steps in and two steps out), which comes out to around 45 breaths per minute. If you are using the talk test, you should be able to say a sentence or two, but that's really it. If you can recite the plot of the last movie you saw on Netflix, that's not a tempo.

Even for experienced runners, figuring out your tempo pace is something that you will have to continue to tweak. Your pace will depend on conditions, and it's very easy to let your ego get in the way of a good run.

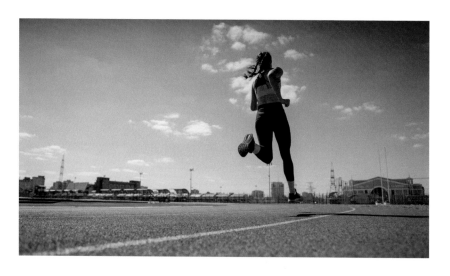

Speed Workouts or VO2max

These can be a lot of fun, or they can be terrifying for a new runner. The goal with a speed workout is to run hard, but to PACE yourself. You don't want to run the first few intervals so hard that you collapse before the workout is done. Every workout will feel harder the longer it goes, so in order to get even pacing from the beginning, you need to sandbag the first few, keep it controlled in the middle, and then give it just about all you've got at the end.

From a pacing perspective, VO2max workouts are completed at 5k pace or faster, sometimes much faster! So what's the reason behind these workouts (besides just getting faster)?

Defined simply, VO2max is the maximum amount of oxygen your body can utilize during exercise. It's a combination of how much oxygen-rich blood your heart can pump and the muscles' ability to use that oxygen.

Training at VO2max increases the amount of oxygen your body can use. The more oxygen you can use, the faster you can run. (Well, for the most part, but let's keep it simple here). Besides boosting your ability to use oxygen, speed workouts force you to run more efficiently and with better form to hit those speedy times. That will translate to better form at all speeds.

What Does a VO2max Workout Feel Like?

It should feel very hard, but just a smidge under all-out effort. You should be breathing very hard and be very thankful when you get to the end of each interval. At the end of the whole workout, you should think that you could maybe run one or two more intervals, but you wouldn't want to.

Most runners use a 1:2 or a 2:1 ratio breathing rhythm. This works out to be about 60 breaths per minute. And the talk test? Maybe you can get out a word or two, but that's about it.

Now, you should be running hard, but not quite so hard that you are doubling over at the end of each rep with your hands on your knees. That's when you know you should take it down a notch.

What something feels like in perfect weather is not going to feel the same in heat or cold or on hills or on days where you just had a fight with your spouse. Those days are going to feel harder, so the body will get a tough workout at a slower pace.

Pace Perfection is an Illusion

Hopefully I've given you some tips to make the most of your workouts. But what I don't want to do is make you feel like every run has to be at the perfect effort level or perfect pace to be effective. It doesn't. All running will make you a better runner, and aiming to at least get in the ballpark with your speed workouts is far more important than stressing out over this pace or that pace.

While it's great to look at each individual workout, sometimes it is also helpful to zoom out to the bigger picture, especially if you are training for a big goal race. Running and training is a journey. It's not always going to be perfect, but you are still getting fitter, and every run contributes to that in its own way.

We always want our hard work to have great results on that big goal day. While we can't guarantee we will get those results every time, making smart choices with your training and learning to feel your training paces will set you up for a much better chance of that happening.

How to Rest Between Intervals

First and foremost to running any workout at any pace is to understand what you are doing and why. All running is good for you, but there truly is a method to the madness when coming up with a smart training program with workouts matched to achieve your goals.

It's easy to think that the fast part of your speed workout is the main objective. The truth is that the rest in between the fast running is just as important.

Endurance and Stamina

For long distance runners, we have two primary objectives. We want to run far and we want to run fast. Your speed is how fast you can run, and your ability to run far is your endurance, but what we really want is the combination of speed and endurance, which is called stamina.

If you are training for a marathon, it really doesn't matter how fast you can run 100 meters or even a mile if you lack the stamina to hang on to that speed for very long. In other words, raw speed is great, but if you can't control it or keep it going for a long time, we have some work to do.

Building endurance is simple, but that doesn't mean it's easy. To be able to run a long time, your lungs have to be able to take in oxygen, which travels through your bloodstream to your muscles, which use it to process energy in the cells. The more often you run aerobically, which means "with oxygen," the better and more efficiently this process works. Aerobic running is long, slow, easy running where you are comfortable and can talk easily with a friend or sing along to the show tunes in your headphones.

Aerobic running is so important to building endurance that it's recommended that 80 percent of the running you do all week is in the easy zone. Not only does it build a huge aerobic engine, but all the time on your feet prepares the legs by gradually and safely building up the muscles, tendons, and bones. Powerful lungs are great, but if you don't take the time required to build up the legs, you're not going to get very far.

Can you run a marathon by only training with easy running? You absolutely can. And if just finishing one is your goal, keeping it easy can be a good way to get to the finish line injury free.

But most runners want to get from point A to point B a little faster than they did last time, or they want to beat their little brother's time, or they want to be able to say they ran a marathon faster than Oprah. Whatever your motivation is, to get faster, you need to run faster.

Remember that when we speed up, we are only trying to do two things: run fast and run far fast. Some workouts are designed to develop your raw speed, while other workouts are meant to boost your stamina.

And if you can figure out which of those goals your workout is preparing you for, you can figure out how to rest.

Speed Development

Speed development workouts tend to be shorter, faster segments with longer rests. The goal is to teach your brain to tell your legs to move quicker than before. It takes a lot of power and energy to run just about as hard as you can for a short period of time, and if you are trying to touch the highest end of your raw speed, getting in a full recovery between sets allows you to maintain your pace over multiple intervals.

A speed development workout could be something like 200-meter repeats where you charge a half lap around the track and come to a standing stop as you catch your breath. If you are bent over at the waist with your hands on your knees, that's a good sign that you went too hard, but occasionally that will happen on these kinds of workouts. If it happens every rep, you'll want to slow down the remaining fast segments to a more controllable pace; if you don't, your exhaustion will force you to slow down anyway. Far better to drive the bus yourself than let fatigue or injury take the wheel.

In just about any workout, we are looking for challenging but doable, so if you have started out so hard that your rests get longer and your speed sections get slower, that's a sign to pull back and sometimes means you should start your cool-down. Even splits on both the rests and the intervals is the ideal goal because it shows that you understand how to pace yourself, which is essential to racing well. Pacing is a skill that takes time to learn, so don't get too caught up worrying about perfectly even splits.

In general, if the workout is designed to touch the top end of your speed at a given distance, whether it's a 200 or a set of mile repeats, we want the rests to allow you enough recovery so that you can repeat the effort just as well the first time as the last time. If that means you walk, that's just fine.

Stamina Workouts Should Be Continuous

For workouts that are designed to build your stamina, the spirit of the workout will be better achieved if you jog the rests instead of stopping to walk, unless you have to. Typically those workouts involve longer intervals of perhaps two miles with jogs in between, but it doesn't have to be that way.

One of my favorite stamina-building workouts is an alternating 200-meter workout. Unlike the sprinting 200-meter workout I just talked about, the alternating 200

SHOULD YOU JOG OR WALK YOUR INTERVAL RECOVERIES?

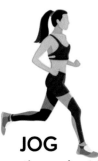 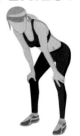

JOG

- allows the workout to be continuous, which builds stamina
- keeps the blood flowing, clearing waste products more efficiently
- does not allow fastest intervals possible
- perceived effort is harder without complete rest

STAND OR WALK

- allows fastest intervals possible
- more time spent in highest VO2 max zone, developing high end speed
- waste products build higher which trains you to cope and still run hard
- perceived effort is easier with complete rest

the planted *runner*

switches between a fast 200 and a recovery jog 200, but it goes on for miles and miles, depending on the ability of the athlete and the race they are training for. The key is understanding how to rest here is that the fast 200s are not going to be anywhere near the pace you could sprint a 200—it's more like your 5k race pace—so you can jog the recovery 200s at a much faster jog than you could between sprint intervals. What's great about this workout is that you can run the equivalent of a 5k race at your race pace, while the jogging in between keeps the effort aerobic, and you won't be wrecked for the rest of the day like you would after a really hard 5k race effort.

In other words, continuous effort, or jogging the rests, is more important for building stamina, while full recovery, or stopping and walking, is more appropriate for improving your raw speed.

Done Is Better Than Perfect

All that being said, we don't live in a perfect world, and some days are harder than others for lots of reasons that have nothing to do with running. You could start out a stamina workout with every intention of jogging the rests, and by the eighth interval, you need to walk. That is perfectly fine! Walk, regroup, and get back at it. The workout is not ruined and you are not a failure; you are still working hard and improving your skills.

Many times, you can recover enough to get right back where you want to be. Other times, a workout will go south, and no matter how you rest, the wheels fly off the train and you can't get back on. You can try again, but if your form is falling apart and you can't get anywhere close to where you need to be, that's a sign to go ahead and cool down. One workout isn't going to make or break you, unless you don't learn from it.

The most important takeaway is that you should value the rest as much as the running and try to be as consistent with those as you can. Once you understand the reason why you are running what you are running, you can get the most benefit out of the workout and eventually get from Point A to Point B faster than you ever could before.

Hills Are Strength and Speed in Disguise

Want to build better legs? You know, tough, durable legs that can tackle anything without getting beat up? Sprinkle in some hills.

I live on a ridge in the mountains. So unless I want to run back and forth on the same two mile flat stretch (which I often do), hills are a part of every run. But I have to be honest. Sometimes, I want to avoid hills. Running is hard enough without being forced to fight gravity! But learning to embrace hills can make you a stronger, more durable runner.

That's because hill running is strength training in disguise. It builds muscle in your calves, quads, hamstrings, and glutes. You'll also strengthen your hip flexors and Achilles' tendons more than you can on perfectly flat ground.

And building strength is just one of the benefits of hills. You'll also boost your speed, endurance, and perhaps even your confidence if you add some elevation to your runs.

How to Run Hills

The two most important parts of running hills well is great form and great mental attitude. Proper form will help you conquer the hill with less effort, and embracing the hill mentally will enable you to reach the top with far less struggle.

In order to run with great form uphill, it can help to visualize what that looks like first. The most important element is that you keep your chest up and your shoulders down and back. This allows your lungs to fully expand and take in as much oxygen as possible.

Many times, runners will encounter a hill and will unconsciously hunch forward, unknowingly constricting their airway. Whether this is a physical manifestation of a mental struggle about being forced to work harder or not, crouching forward will make the hill more difficult.

Instead, keep your head and eyes up, looking in front of you instead of looking down. Pretend that you are wearing a name tag on your chest and you want everyone ahead to see it!

You want to lean into the hill, but not at the waist. It's better to feel the lean coming from your ankles. If you were to stop and stand still, you should be leaning enough to fall forward.

Your arms should be bent at about 90-degree angles at the elbow. Use the power of your arms to help drive the legs forward, not across the body. After all, what your arms do, your legs will do, so keep them active.

To gain power, drive your knee up and off the hill, not straight ahead into the hill. This is slightly different from a good knee drive on flat ground where the knee tracks straight ahead.

Of course, your power is not actually coming from the knees on hills. Your hips and your glutes are pushing your legs up and forward. I find it helps to think about the working muscles when you are running uphill to make sure those big muscles are

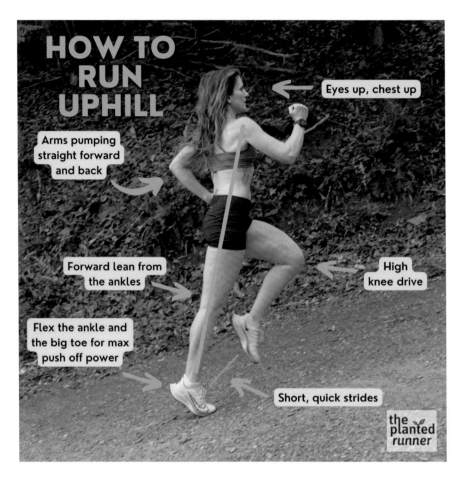

doing the work instead of the smaller calf muscles. It is nearly impossible to land on your heel when running up a hill. This is part of why running up hills can be so helpful to improving your form. If you tend to overstride, adding hills to your runs can help you kick the habit.

Your ankles and your feet also get in on the action, springing you up and forward. When you dorsiflex your ankle, or point your toes towards the ground, it helps push you off the ground. Your big toe is the same. Aiming to get the most extension possible from both the ankle and the big toe can make a big difference in how efficient you are with each stride. The more efficient you are, the easier you can run with less energy.

Hill Sprints

Mixing hills into a run is a great way to add challenge and build strength, but if you want to truly maximize all the benefits of hills, try some specific hill workouts. Hill repeats can be done as their own workout, or you can swap out your flatland strides for a few hill strides after an easy run (see the Strides section in chapter five).

For hill repeats, plan to be at the bottom of a runnable hill after a 15- to 20-minute jogging warm-up. The hill should be a real hill but not so steep that you have to hike up it (about four to six percent incline is perfect if you are doing this on a treadmill).

To begin, run up the hill at a hard but controlled effort, focusing on all the good form cues that I just mentioned. After 60 seconds, come to a stop and note where you reached on the hill. Jog or walk back down and rest until your heart rate comes back to near normal. Repeat 4 to 10 times, depending on your fitness level, aiming to hit the same spot on the hill as you did the first time.

While you are trying to run fast, speed is not the ultimate goal with hill repeats. You will always be slower on uphills than you are on flat ground, so hill workouts are always about effort, not pace.

Even with perfect form, uphill running can be harder on runners that are prone to lower leg injuries like calf and Achilles issues. But if you are healthy, hills can be a great way to build strength and speed and improve your form on any surface.

How Downhill Running Builds Better Legs

Now that you know running up hills is good for you, what about the other half, running down hills? Most runners think about the uphill being the hard part. But if you really want to build better legs, working on downhills can be just as beneficial.

Why Downhill? Isn't That the Easy Part?

The thing that I love most about downhill running is that it's fun! You can fly down a hill with less effort and at faster speeds than you can on flat land, and it really makes you feel like a little kid without a care in the world. Your lungs do not have to work as hard, and your legs can turn over just about as quickly as they can.

More and more people are seeking out downhill races because they think they will have a better chance of a faster finishing time if they can just fly downhill. While for many people that is the case, for others, a downhill course can absolutely wreck them.

And if you're a trail runner, hills are just part of the deal. Many trail runners are actually SLOWER on technical downhills because they lack the confidence that rock-solid quads and good technique give you.

There is a technique to running downhill and definitely some things you want to keep in mind about training and racing downhill. If you do it right, you can take advantage of gravity's free speed, but if you do it wrong, you can send much stronger shock waves up your legs and burn out your quads, risking both performance and injury.

So How Do You Do It?

Just like when running uphill, you want to have a slight lean forward at the hips to take advantage of the downhill. Don't overdo the lean; you only need a slight tilt to benefit from gravity.

Now this is going to feel really awkward at first. Our natural human instinct is to lean back into the hill to prevent ourselves from tumbling all the way down and crashing. But what happens when we lean back is that our foot goes forward ahead of us, and often the heel hits the ground first. There's nothing inherently wrong with heel striking, but if your foot hits the ground before your center of gravity crosses above it, you are adding pounds more stress to your legs. Not only that, but you are braking with every step, giving up the free energy that the downhill is supposed to give you. So you are increasing your chance for injury as well as slowing yourself down at the same time. Not a great idea.

But if you lean down the hill slightly, gravity will pull you forward, so you will have to work less. If you think of downhill running as controlled falling, you can capture that energy and use it for speed. Again, we have an instinct to avoid falling, so this might feel a little strange and even scary on certain hills, but the more you practice it, the better at it you'll get.

Remember: Lean forward to avoid braking and breaking!

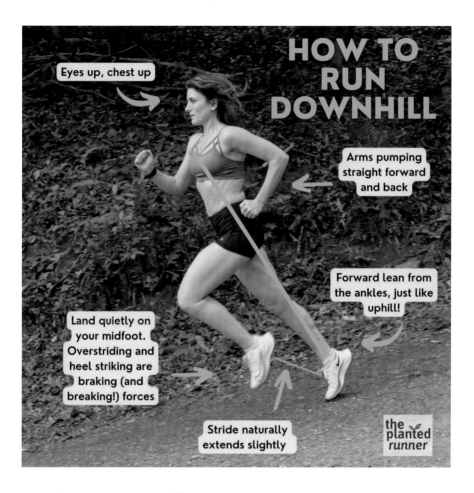

So What Do You Do With Your Arms?

For a road race or another smooth surface, you want to keep your arms relaxed and only slightly moving forward and back. You don't want to flail them out to the sides because it wastes energy.

On the other hand, for a technical trail race where you are maneuvering over roots and rocks and uneven surfaces, using your arms for balance can be a very good thing. The little energy that it costs to use your arms can be a small investment if it prevents a tumble down the trail.

On the roads where you are not expecting any obstacles, keep your head up and your eyes looking forward instead of down. This is also something that might not feel natural right away, because when we are afraid of falling, we want to look down. Don't do that. Look ahead to where you are going, not where your feet are.

On trails, of course, you will need to shorten your gaze to avoid obstacles, but you still should be looking several feet ahead of you and not down at your feet.

Getting good at the forward lean takes practice, but eventually you will build confidence. Confidently leaning forward when your instinct is to pull back will not be automatic, so practice it every time you go downhill.

What About Your Feet?

You'll want to land with your foot right beneath your torso or as close as you can. Depending on the grade of the downhill, you might not quite land underneath your torso, and that's okay if it's not too much. In general, the steeper the grade, the more likely your foot is to land out in front.

Again, when you extend your leg too much ahead of the rest of your body, you are more likely to land on your heel, which will act like a braking motion. Focus on landing towards your midfoot to maintain speed while staying in control.

You will notice that your stride length naturally extends when running downhill. However, you should not try to consciously increase your stride length. Let the grade of the hill do this naturally for you.

Aren't Downhills Bad for My Knees?

Running hard downhill is eccentric muscle training, meaning the work is done as the muscle is lengthening. No other form of running will do this.

Downhill running increases your quadricep and hamstring strength and stiffness, improves running efficiency, and has been shown to reduce delayed-onset muscle syndrome.

And of course, it makes you a better downhill runner!

If you are a healthy runner who introduces downhills gradually and recovers adequately, you are not risking your knees but are, in fact, strengthening them. If you have current or recurring knee issues, be even more gentle with downhills;

ultimately, however, the strength gains from downhill running helps support your knees.

Downhill Repeats Workout

- Choose a hill that is fairly steep but not technical if you are on trails. It should be something that you feel comfortable running down quickly, and the grade will depend on your ability.
- After you've run your usual warm-up mile or two, jog up the hill for about a minute or so. Remember the up is the rest and the down is the work, so be sure to jog the ups. At the top, stop and catch your breath for as long as you need to, usually 30 to 60 seconds.
- Then get ready to rip! Fly down that hill as fast as you feel comfortable using great technique. The length of your hill is determined by your ability, but most runners should take 30 to 45 seconds or so to get down.
- Stand at the bottom for 30 to 60 seconds to catch your breath and then repeat 6 to 10 times, depending on your ability.
- Run your usual cool-down of a mile or two.

If you've never done this kind of downhill training, be warned: THIS IS EXTREMELY TOUGH, AND YOU WILL BE SORE! So go easier than feels necessary at first. You can add these in once a month to start and then progress up to every other week.

What's the Best Way to Race Downhill?

The answer is a bit course dependent.

Let's look at the iconic downhill course, the Boston Marathon. Boston is a net downhill course, dropping 447 feet/136 meters over the course of the full 42.2k distance. But it actually has the slowest time of all the majors if you look at elite finishing times. One of the main reasons for that is the series of uphills at the 20-mile mark as well as the relatively high chance of fighting a headwind. But nonetheless, just because it's a net downhill, does not mean it's fast.

The general strategy for running Boston is to avoid getting too carried away with your speed on the first 20 miles of descent, because if you burn up your quads, Heartbreak Hill will feel like Mount Everest. And even if you manage to crest the hills intact, the final six miles downhill of the race will feel like you are running on legs made of wet spaghetti.

Increasing in popularity are the really dramatic downhill races such as the REVEL series of races in the Western US. You are shuttled to the top of a mountain and basically roll down the hill to the finish line. These are fun, and they are fast, but if you have not properly toughened up your quads with lots of downhills in training, you might find these types of races to be exceptionally painful.

Besides Training on Downhills What Else Can You Do?

Toughen up those quads in the gym. Wall sits, where you press your back into the wall as you squat (it looks like you are sitting in a chair without the chair) are a great option. Take your wall sit up a notch by holding a weight or lifting your heels into a calf raise. Lunges of all kinds, both with weights and without, elevated on a step and on the ground, are all good quad strengtheners.

Another tip, especially if you don't have a lot of downhills to train on, is to use a downhill treadmill or elevate the back of a treadmill to make a decline. Be sure to get the okay with your gym before you do this if you don't have a treadmill at home! This way, you can train on the decline without ever going outside.

Just remember that a little goes a long way. You don't need all your runs to be on a downhill to get good at them. Two or three times a week is usually plenty. As you get closer to the race, you'll want to make sure that you do at least two point to point long runs on a decline if you can.

With practice and good technique, you can learn to run and race downhill safely and effectively, and who knows? You might even have some fun.

Two Most Common Causes of Injuries for Runners

Depending on the data you look at, anywhere from 50 to 70 percent of runners will get injured this year. And probably closer to 99 percent of runners will get injured at some point in their running lifetime.

Runners get hurt. They get hurt a lot. There are several specific ways that runners get hurt, but there are two that are the most common. Thankfully, they are also largely preventable. And it all relates to speed.

Running Too Fast Is a Recipe for Injury

The two most common ways runners get injured are running easy days too fast and running workout days too fast.

We runners love to see progress and love to run fast when we feel good. Once you are beyond the beginning stage when all things running are hard and everything hurts, running is actually fun sometimes! And running fast? That's really fun. Especially when you look at your watch and you've never gone this fast, this long before. It's awesome.

You get a runner's high just knowing that you ran faster than you did yesterday because all the things that suck about running like the hard work and the discipline are instantly forgotten and you just get to feel awesome and happy about what a badass you are.

So you do it again the next day. And that feels great, too! Well, your calf feels a little tight, but so what? You are NAILING your 400-meter repeats today. Running is the best thing ever!

And you do it over and over again, not necessarily pushing every day to the top of your ability, but your easy runs gradually get faster and your drive to hit your workout splits to get that dopamine-laced shot of accomplishment increases little by little.

Then maybe, out of nowhere, you are sidelined with an injury. Maybe you were out on an easy run and felt a twinge in your knee. Or maybe you were on the track and felt a sharp pull in your hamstring.

You might be tempted to blame that one workout for your injury, but the truth is the seeds were sown for that to happen much, much earlier. Every time we run too fast, even by a few seconds, we are adding a straw to the camel's back. You might not get injured immediately, but those straws add up day after day.

Running Easy Days Too Fast

Let's start with easy day running. Easy needs to be easy, no matter what the terrain or the weather. If it helps, think of your easy days as just practice running. You are jogging. Embrace the jog!

Easy runs are designed to be so easy that they don't require recovery for themselves. If you push the pace, you will require more recovery, which means your speed days can't be as good because you are not 100 percent ready. That means you will be slower when you want to be fast, which means it will take longer to improve.

Yes, it's a paradox that running slower will make you faster, but it's because you will feel and perform better on the days where speed matters.

Eventually, most runners grow to accept the "easy days easy" and "hard days hard" concept.

Running Speed Days Too Fast

Why shouldn't you run faster on a workout day? After all, that's where you are given permission to finally go fast after jogging all week! If you can run faster on speed days, doesn't that mean you are improving?

The thing is, on most workout days, you should KNOW that you can run faster. But you are CHOOSING not to.

I know, this sounds crazy, right?

But you do not PROVE your fitness on training days. That is where you BUILD your fitness.

Building fitness is best done in small, controlled increments. So small that your body easily adapts without sending off the alarm that major damage is occurring.

Because that's what happens when you run hard. You are damaging the fibers in your muscles on purpose so that your body can go in and build you back stronger than before. But if you do it too fast, instead of getting small micro-tears, we are creating more serious damage that is more difficult to repair quickly.

When you build gradually with patience, your body can handle it. You slightly damage your tissues, and when you rest, the cleanup and repair crew in your cells heads in and fixes you up better than you were before.

Before you know it, you are fitter and stronger and injury free.

So if you are running your workouts so hard that it takes an all-out effort, you are dramatically increasing your risk of injury. This is not to say that you should be lazy and not work hard. You should absolutely work hard on your hard days. But there is a difference between running relaxed and under control while still running fast, versus straining and reaching and stressing and giving it everything you've got every single time.

And when you are just starting out, it's not as easy to tell where that line between good effort and extraordinary effort is; that takes some trial and error. But I'd rather have you err on the side of not quite hard enough than so hard that you can't run at all.

Running too fast on your easy days and running too fast on your workout days are not the only causes of running injuries, but they are two main culprits, and they are preventable.

So take it down just a notch so that you can hopefully be one of the 30 percent of runners that stays injury free this year.

Train Your Tummy: Tips for a Happy Running Belly

It's no secret that running can be pretty rough on the stomach. There are few runners that have never experienced at least a little gastric distress on the run. The good news is that just like your leg muscles, the stomach can be trained to be able to handle the rigors of running without getting sick.

The Causes of Stomach Issues on the Run

As you run, your body decides that you must be running away from a saber tooth tiger or chasing down a water buffalo for dinner, so digestion on the run becomes less of a priority. The blood that normally goes to the stomach and gut instead gets diverted to the working muscles to power your run.

So whatever is left in your stomach gets bounced around and digests much more slowly than it would be if you were lying on the couch. All that bouncing on a full or even partially full stomach can cause that uncomfortable feeling in your tummy.

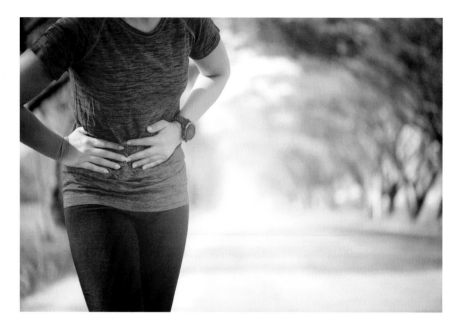

Not every runner's system reacts the same way, so you and your running buddy might experience different symptoms even with the same breakfast on the same run. Some runners have more upper digestive symptoms, such as burping, reflux, nausea, or even vomiting, while others have mid- or lower-intestinal pain, which can lead to a very uncomfortable run and unexpected port-a-potty stops.

Therefore, runners need to learn what kinds of foods cause trouble on the run and what kind of timing of meals before runs work best to keep the belly happy.

It's pretty obvious that downing a burger and extra-large fries immediately before a run is a high-risk idea, but there are other culprits that might take a little experimenting to discover.

Dehydration and Overhydration

The first problem could be dehydration. If you are not properly hydrated, especially when running in warm weather, your stomach complaining might be the first sign. Remember that running causes blood to flow away from the stomach, so if you are beginning the run dehydrated, it will just get worse as you run.

But the opposite issue can cause problems, too. If you are overhydrated, the sloshing of liquid in your belly can be very painful, so make sure that you sip instead of chug, and don't drink too much. This can be a big issue in long races like the marathon, when runners try to stick to a predetermined hydration schedule that's not based on what is actually happening in the moment. If your stomach feels like a water balloon, stop drinking!

Too Much Food

Just as too much fluid is a problem, the same goes with too much food. A normal sized meal will take two to three hours to digest properly, so be sure that you are not running right after a big meal. But you don't want to run totally empty, especially when you have a long run or big workout, so I recommend finding an easy to digest food that you can eat in the hour before a run.

Popular choices are bananas, dates, a little juice, or some crackers. Having a go-to food can be really helpful on race day to pre-fuel your race, without getting full or having too much jostling in your stomach.

Gels and New Fuels

The next culprit could be trying something new before or during a run. That new gel that your friend uses or the latest energy bar might be a nice change if you always eat the same thing, but it can be an unwelcome surprise on your belly. So stick with what works, until it doesn't!

Speaking of gels, they, along with popular sports drinks, are notorious for causing GI issues, especially late in a race. The reason they work so well is that the sugar moves quickly through to the bloodstream, but if you don't train your stomach to handle it, you might find yourself too sick to take in any more calories by mile 16. So be sure to train often with what you will use on race day to be sure what flavors and brands work for you.

Fiber, Fat, and Protein

While too much sugar can be an issue, too much protein, fat, and fiber could also lead to trouble. These nutrients take longer to digest, so if they are still in your system during your run, your body might decide it wants to eject them as soon as possible. I'm not saying you should eliminate healthy foods in your diet, but watch how closely you eat fiber before a run.

Feeling Sick After the Run

What if you don't typically feel sick on the run, but the thought of food after a run turns your stomach? You know that you need to get in recovery foods, but they are really hard to stomach for you right away.

The first thing to know is that you don't have to force feed yourself right after a run. The idea that there is a very tight recovery window has largely been discounted by recent research, so try to at least get in a few sips of water immediately and then shower and relax a little until your appetite comes back.

You obviously don't want to wait the entire day before eating again, but an hour or two isn't going to make much difference. It's far better to eat real, whole foods when you are ready instead of forcing down a highly processed protein concoction just because you are trying to hit some magic recovery window that really doesn't exist.

Next Steps

If you have tried everything I've mentioned and are still having issues, I suggest you get very detailed and start logging your food to see if you can find any clues. You could have an undiagnosed food allergy or intolerance, or you could have a chronic medical condition like celiac disease or irritable bowel syndrome. Those conditions typically include symptoms other than just feeling sick on the run, so keep a journal of when you are feeling off to see if you can make a connection.

Like almost everything running, you have to experiment with what works for you, and once you find something that seems to work, stick with it as much as you can. Because running is supposed to be good for you, not make you sick.

Chapter Six

Strength, Balance, and Mobility Training for Runners

Simple routines to keep you strong, balanced, and injury free

Strength Training for Runners

Strength training for runners doesn't have to take a lot of time. And the results are worth the investment!

If you want to become a better runner, the first place to start is to run a little bit more. That could mean lengthening your runs or adding in another day per week. But there will come a point where you simply can't (and shouldn't!) run more.

And that's where strength training comes in.

Why Runners Should Strength Train

The two main benefits of strength training for runners are that it prevents and helps heal injuries, and it enhances performance. Done properly, strength training creates a foundation for injury-free running and allows you to keep increasing mileage and intensity on your runs.

And on the performance side, studies have shown that resistance training improves running economy and endurance muscle fibers. Research has also linked weight training to better body composition and resting metabolic rates.

Not to mention, strength training is particularly important as we get older in a way that running alone is not. Recent studies have proven that running does not protect against the gradual loss of lean muscle tissue, and, as we lose muscle, we also lose a larger percentage of our fast-twitch muscle fibers, which is part of why we slow down as we age.

To say it another way, if you are afraid of getting slower as you get older, making strength training a part of your routine will slow down that slow down.

To be clear, endurance runners do not need to be super strong and muscular. Just take a look at the difference between a 100-meter sprinter's body and an elite marathoner. The sprinter will be visibly muscular, and the marathoner will be much leaner. That's because sprinting requires huge explosive power from big muscles while endurance runners simply need to be strong enough to endure mile after mile.

The good news is that if you are an endurance runner, you don't have to spend as much time lifting weights as a sprinter would. And you don't have to attack your strength sessions with the same amount of discipline and focus as you do your speed days on the track.

The thing to remember is that if running is your primary focus, your strength work should complement your running, not compete with it.

When to Strength Train

The timing of your gym sessions is important. If you are lifting twice a week, you do not want to be doing that on your easy days. Easy days are meant for recovery from your harder runs, not for additional muscle damage from lifting weights, even if you are lifting light. The absolute best way to complement your running is to lift on the same day as your hardest runs.

In other words, you want your hard days to be hard, and your easy days to be easy.

The reason you want to be doing your heavy lifting on the same days as your fast running is because this allows your easy and rest days to be truly restorative. We don't build fitness when we work out; we build when the body is given time to repair.

If you run hard at the track on Tuesday, lift weights on Wednesday, then do your fast-tempo run on Thursday, your body has very little time to repair the damage between workouts. Not only will you likely feel sore most of the time and run slower when you are trying to run fast, you are diminishing the effectiveness of all three of the workouts.

The thing to remember is that you want your strength training to enhance your running, not take away from it, so you need to time it so that you are fresh for running fast and tired for lifting weights. And you don't need to spend an entire hour lifting. A little goes a long way.

Lifting while being a little sore or tired from a hard running workout means that it's tougher to overdo it in the gym, which means that it's easier to recover from both the fast running and the lifting. Scheduling an easy run after strength training also helps ensure that your easy run is appropriately easy, because again, you are a little tired from lifting, so running slower is easier to do.

If you run truly easy on your easy days, you need very little recovery time and will be fresh enough to run to your potential on the fast days, therefore getting a better running workout in.

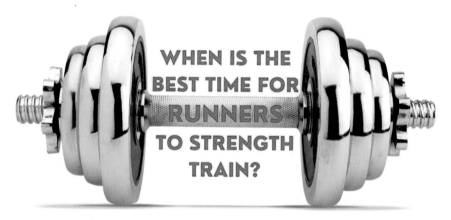

WHEN IS THE BEST TIME FOR RUNNERS TO STRENGTH TRAIN?

STRENGTH TRAIN ON YOUR HARDEST RUNNING DAYS:
This seems counterintuitive, but this ensures that your hard days are truly hard and recovery days are truly easy.

FIRST PRIORITY GOES FIRST:
If running is your main goal, run first, then lift. This way, you are fresh to run well, but if you are tired for strength training, that's less important.

DONE IS BETTER THAN PERFECT:
Squeeze in strength sessions whenever it works for you!

the planted *runner*

How Much Strength Training You Need

Most long-distance runners only need to strength train about 30 to 60 minutes a week. That can be 10 minutes a day or two days of 20 to 30 minutes a week. A little really does go a long way, but once a week is probably not often enough.

If you are crunched for time, one great option is to chop 10 minutes off your daily runs and spend 10 minutes strength training every day. Over the course of a week, that's 70 minutes of strength training, which is awesome, but you are breaking it up into such small chunks that you don't need much recovery.

Perhaps on Monday, instead of running 40 minutes, you run 30 and do some core work like planks, crunches, and bicycles. On Tuesday, you shorten your speed session a little, cool down with some easy jogging, and do some lunges, squats, and calf raises. Wednesday could be upper body. Repeat the pattern for the rest of the week, and include a full rest day.

For those runners who prefer to do longer sessions two or three times a week, it's best to follow those either immediately after your hard or long runs or a few hours later.

For example, if you have a tempo run in the morning, follow it by a 20- to 30-minute strength workout at noon or in the evening. That way, you are adding to the training effect of the running, then fully recovering from both on the following easy days.

The Four Best Strength-Training Exercises for Runners

The four best exercises for runners are squats, deadlifts, lunges, and planks. These exercises can be done anywhere, you can do them with just your body weight or with dumbbells, and there are plenty of variations to keep things interesting.

Let's break each down.

Squats

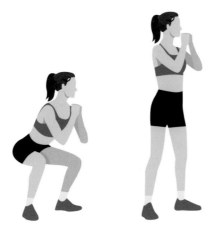

In a standard bodyweight squat, you are targeting your quads, hamstrings, glutes, abdominals, and calves, which are all essential to good running. You can add variation by lifting one heel to weight one leg more than the other, open your stance and target your inner thighs and do a sumo squat, or add a jump to make the move more powerful.

Lunges

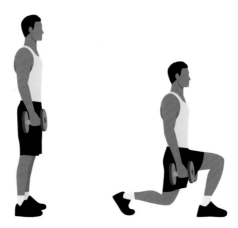

Lunges also work the quads, glutes, hamstrings, and calves as well as other supporting leg muscles, depending on the angle you perform them on. Forwards, backwards, laterally, or adding a torso twist are all great variations.

Deadlifts

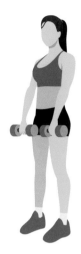
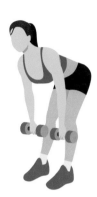

A deadlift is another compound exercise where, traditionally, a weighted barbell starts on the floor. Since you lift it with no momentum, you are lifting "dead weight," which gives the exercise its name.

Deadlifts train multiple muscle groups including the hamstrings, glutes, back, hips, and core.

When it comes to strength training, some people believe that you should really focus on your legs, because that's what you use for running. Other people think you can go light on the legs, because running strengthens those, so you should focus on the core. And many runners simply have no idea what to do with their arms.

Research on runners makes it clear that upper-body, lower-body, and core strength training all contribute to improved running performance. So yeah, that's just about everything. You should do exercises that involve all of the major muscle groups, because that helps create balance as everything is connected.

A slightly different variation is the Romanian deadlift, which focuses more on the hamstrings. You start with a bar or a set of dumbbells at your hip level with your palms facing down. Keep the weights close to your body as you lower it toward your feet, pushing your hips back throughout the movement. Your legs should have a slight bend in the knees. Drive your hips forward to stand up tall, keeping the barbell or dumbbells in front of the thighs.

Plank

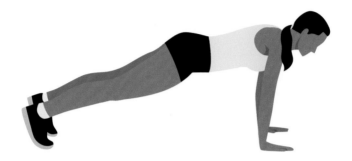

The last of my four favorite strength training moves for runners is the plank. Planks are amazing because they truly are a full body exercise with plenty of ways to mix them up.

It's named plank for a very good reason: You should look like a board with no bends. You want your body from the tip of your head down to your heels to be in a perfectly straight line. Common mistakes are pushing your booty in the air or letting your hips sag toward the ground.

To do them right, keep your core engaged, maintain a neutral spine, and be sure to breathe.

Plank can either be done in push up position, with your arms locked straight, or you can rest on your forearms. If you are not strong enough to stay up on your toes, use a bench or a set of stairs to elevate your arms a bit higher.

Try to resist the temptation to do plank on your knees, because it's not putting you in proper alignment. If you are still not strong enough to hold plank on an elevated platform or stair without going to your knees, use the wall instead. Once you build strength, you can work your way down to the floor.

If you've never done plank before, aim for 20 to 30 seconds. Advanced runners can try for two minutes or more.

Other Strength-Training Exercises

Now, just because I love those four exercises as well as their million variations, it doesn't mean you are limited to just those, though they are a great foundation. Moving your muscles against resistance can be achieved with your body weight, a resistance band, a machine, or with free weights—your muscles don't know the difference.

I would argue, however, that machines at the gym do take away the work of the stabilizing muscles, which means you get less bang for your strength training buck. For example, if you sit down and do the leg press, there is no need to counterbalance or engage your core. And that means you'll have to do another exercise to target the core.

Now, when I say "core," do you automatically think sit ups and crunches? Those are great if your goal is to look strong, but to actually get a strong core, there's a much better way. And that's unilateral training.

Unilateral Training

Unilateral training is lifting a weight on only one side of the body at a time. Lunges are unilateral because you are doing one leg at a time. Standard squats, where both legs are planted equally on the floor, are bilateral.

But if you lift one heel while doing a squat or hold a dumbbell in just one hand, one side of your body has to do more work. Your core is forced to engage to keep you from falling over. So by lifting unilaterally, you are sneaking in the core stabilizing work runners need without doing a single sit up.

Lift Slow and Heavy

Alright, so you've chosen what to lift, but how heavy should you go, and how many reps should you do? Actually, the number of reps is not critically important. The gym is not where you work on your endurance. You do that on the run. Recent research has shown that doing 5 reps or 20 reps will produce the same benefit in terms of muscle strength and endurance. That's important for busy runners.

Some runners believe that they should only do bodyweight work because it's easier and runners don't really need to bulk up. Well, just because it's body weight doesn't mean it's easy! Pull ups, for example, are extremely challenging for most people, even though it's just bodyweight.

What's more important than the number of times you lift a weight is how you lift them. It's far more effective to lift and lower the weight slowly. Take two to three seconds to lift the weight and at least three seconds to lower the weight, pausing at the hardest point for a second before you lift again.

The reason for the slow lift is you want to eliminate momentum. Momentum cheats your muscles, because the swing is doing the work for you. In addition, the faster you move, the greater the force on your joints and connective tissue, which means the greater the risk for injury. Lifting weights too quickly is far tougher on the joints than lifting too heavy.

Power Boost at the End

If you are looking for a power boost, save your explosive effort for the end of each set of exercises, when you are getting fatigued. Fast movement will be impossible at this point, which protects you from its risks. But from a muscle fiber recruitment standpoint, it still is fast-twitch training. This type of strength training for runners is safer than plyometric exercises and produces the same powerful effects.

You'll want to lift a weight heavy enough to fatigue the muscle you are working within 8 to 20 reps. You'll know when to stop when it is impossible to complete one more with perfect form. This ensures that the muscle fiber is being completely recruited during each and every lift.

Save Time With Fewer Heavier Reps

Let's do a little math: If you are taking three seconds to lift a weight and three seconds to lower it, with a pause in the middle, that's seven seconds per rep. If you choose a weight heavy enough to exhaust you in eight reps, that's 56 seconds per muscle group. If you divide the body into five major muscle groups (chest, back, arms and shoulders, abdominals or core, and legs and glutes), that means you can work every part of your body in about five minutes. Add in some time to rest between sets, and you're done in 10 minutes.

If you have more time and prefer lifting lighter weights with more reps, by all means go for it, but remember, you are not running and don't want to turn your gym session into anything aerobic. A better use of your time would be adding in different exercises. So instead of doing 20 hamstring curls, for example, do just 10 to fatigue, and then do 10 heavy calf raises to fatigue.

Consistency Over Intensity

When in doubt, less is more when it comes to strength training for runners, as long as you consistently do it a few times a week.

So there you have it. A little strength training for runners, a few days a week, mainly after your harder runs, with compound exercises like squats, lunges, deadlifts, and planks, is the magic formula. Well, it's not magic, but it's an investment.

An investment that will pay off by making you a more durable, faster runner, not to mention slow the effects of aging.

The important thing to remember is that no one is perfect, and that's okay. Unless you are a professional runner or can afford to do nothing but work out all the time and at all the perfect times, sometimes you just have to be flexible and do what you can when you can.

But as long as you follow the general rhythm of hard days followed by enough easy days to properly recover, you will maximize all your workouts, spend less time feeling sore, and spend more time running fast and injury free.

Secrets to the Six Pack! (And What to Focus on Instead)

For many people, the idea of getting a flat stomach, or six pack, is one of the reasons to run in the first place. I'm the first to admit that trying to look good at my high school reunion got me back into running in my late 30s. A strong, sexy stomach can be what drives you to get out of bed at four a.m. and go running in the dark every day.

And for some people, it seems like that's all it takes. A little running, a few crunches, and those six-pack abs just seem to appear effortlessly. Well, I'm here to break it to you that for about 95 percent of us (I'm making up that statistic, but I mean pretty much everyone), that's just not going to happen without a whole lot of work and nutritional sacrifice, especially if you are over the age of 25.

Because we all have a six pack in there somewhere, and it's called the rectus abdominus. It's just that the majority of us are not lean enough for those muscles to show, no matter how strong we are. Or, we actually are perfectly lean enough, but the washboard abs don't appear due to genetics. Some people just tend to carry their fat in their bellies, while others stash it away elsewhere.

The body fat percentages needed to see visible abs is a huge range, which actually corresponds to a healthy body composition. For women, that's about 17 to 24 percent, and for men, that's about 6 to 17 percent. If you are at the lower end, you are likely to look more sculpted, but some lucky tummies start looking ripped at the higher end.

Instagram has taught us that a taut tummy with rippling abs is what we all should strive for. And if that's your fitness goal, more power to you.

But I'll let you in on a little secret. Developing a rocking six pack won't do much at all for your running, other than how you look in a sports bra. That's because the rectus abdominis muscles are not particularly useful in the motion of running. They are used for sitting up. Which is why sit ups and crunches are the key to creating great looking abs but are not super helpful for a strong running core.

A Strong Core Isn't Defined by a Six-Pack

If you take a look at the stomachs of elite distance runners, both male and female, you're not always going to see a defined six pack. You'll see lean definition, of course, but only the sprinters have huge muscles. But they all have a strong core.

So what do I mean by core? Your abdominals are certainly a part of the equation, but your hips, glutes, and back muscles also play a big role in making you a better runner.

In running, your legs get all the glory, but you have a strong core to thank for going the distance.

The most efficient distance runners are very stingy with their movements. If a movement is not directly related to propelling you forward, it's wasted energy. So what you want to do is quiet your torso as you run. Your legs and arms move forward and back, but everything directly connected to your spine stays smooth and silent.

In theory, that sounds obvious and easy—just move your arms and legs and don't move anything else. But in reality, you have to tighten your entire torso the whole time to keep it from following your arms and legs. And that takes strength.

On the other hand, if you keep your abs loose and allow your shoulders to relax forward and your head to dip down, you are no longer a tight, efficient spring. You become a wobbly noodle, which is much harder to bounce down the road!

The next reason that we want a strong core is because it holds our torso up in the proper position so the legs and arms can be free to swing. All the muscles in your middle should be taut and contracted as you run so the abs can support the spine in a relatively rigid position. And you can't do that for very long if your core isn't strong enough to support a stable spine.

Here's an analogy: Imagine picking up a little kid who has been told to go limp like a sack of potatoes. It is much harder to do than picking up the same kid who is told to become stiff as a board, because the weight of the limp kid shifts around and is unstable. It's the same with your torso—it's much easier to run with a tight torso and supported spine than a relaxed one.

Runners Need Strong Glutes

While most people don't automatically think of their butt when it comes to the core, it is a key muscle group powering your runs.

Yes, your legs work hard, but if you are relying only on your legs, you are not taking advantage of the biggest muscle in the body, the gluteus maximus (or your butt). Your butt is large and powerful because it has the job of keeping the trunk of the body in an erect posture, preventing the sack of potatoes phenomenon that you often see at the end of a marathon.

But what the glutes can also do is help push your legs forward. Next time you go for a run, think of your legs as the levers and your core (meaning glutes, hips, and abdominal muscles) as the power. Your calf muscles are small and weak compared to your butt, and they are at the wrong end of the lever. If they are doing all the work, you're going to have some serious problems at the end of your race.

Again, you don't need the ripped muscles of a body builder to become more efficient; you just need enough strength to keep your spine stable and aligned and your glutes firing at all times.

No Crunches Necessary

So how do you get a strong core for running? Well, you might have heard that crunches are bad for you or they are not necessary for runners. Or maybe you just guessed that because I just told you that a six pack isn't important. That's all sort of true.

The idea that crunches are bad for you started after a 2001 study that linked crunches to spinal damage. In the study, researchers took pig spines removed from dead pigs and crunched them over and over again thousands of times. Not surprisingly, after tens of thousands of crunches, spinal damage resulted.

Obviously, there are several problems trying to extrapolate these results to humans. You are not a pig, you do not do thousands of crunches a day, and you are not dead. Just like a dead stick will break more easily than a green branch, so will a dead bone versus a living one.

Crunches, which are done by lying on your back with your knees bent and feet flat on the floor and then contracting your abs to slowly lift your shoulder blades off the ground an inch or two, are not bad for you. They will develop those six-pack muscles, if you are lean enough to see them. But they are not the primary spine stabilizers, and they are not attached to your legs, so they don't help your running much at all.

A better use of your time would be planks, of which there are several variations. It could be down on your forearms or up on your hands with locked elbows, side planks, or hip drops—the list of plank variations seems endless.

There are also lots of things you can do from a tabletop position or down on all fours such as balance work like holding the opposite arm and leg out then crunching in or glute and hamstring work by bending and flexing one leg at the knee or drawing circles with your extended leg; all are good choices.

Basically, any move where you use your leg as a lever, whether you're on all fours or your back, will force you to use your core muscles to lift the legs. Just be sure that you are protecting your lower back when you do some of these moves, which can be done by placing your hands or a pillow under your sacrum or lumbar spine for support.

So, if you care more about your splits than a six pack, you never have to do another crunch again.

Mobility and Flexibility

What is mobility? Well, in the simplest terms, it's the ability to move, so obviously everyone who runs has the goal of being more mobile. But we are looking for a little more than that when we run. Mobility is the capacity to actively move a joint through a normal range of motion with efficiency and strength.

Flexibility, on the other hand, is the ability to passively move a joint through a wide range of motion.

To be a better runner, you don't have to be very flexible in most areas. In fact, distance runners are known for being quite inflexible. Eliud Kipchoge, one of the fastest marathoners on earth, famously can't bend down and touch his toes. Clearly, being flexible through the hamstrings is not an issue for him.

In fact, science is showing us that being too flexible might actually hinder your running. The theory is that, like a tightly coiled spring, less flexible hamstrings provide more energy return when you hit the ground, giving you a literal spring in your step.

Runners need to be flexible (have a wide range of motion) in only four places, which I'll go over shortly. But having good mobility through all the joints of the body can help you feel better, run better, recover better, and perhaps even prevent injury.

Both flexibility and mobility can be improved through stretching. But the type of stretching you do matters.

Active Isolated Stretching vs. Static Stretching

Active isolated stretching (AIS) is a type of stretching where you only hold a stretch for two to three seconds at a time. Classic static stretching is where you hold a pose for several seconds or minutes. AIS is better for improving mobility, and static stretching is better for creating more flexibility.

Static Stretching

Let's look at what happens when you stretch statically using the example of the hamstrings or the muscles in the backs of your thighs. There are several ways to stretch the hamstrings, and the simplest one is to just bend over and reach for your toes. If you are very flexible, this might feel easy and good. But if you are not very flexible or you go beyond your natural range of motion, this might feel very uncomfortable and cause pain.

The reason this happens is that when you hold a stretch too far, too fast, or for longer than a couple of seconds, your body starts to try to protect itself from pulling or tearing the muscle. A natural reflex called the myotatic reflex will kick in and try to force you to pull out of the stretch. This happens automatically and ballistically and can cause more harm than good.

Studies have also shown that if you stretch statically before a run on cold muscles, not only can you cause muscle damage, but you can actually decrease your performance on that run. Not a great idea.

If you are going to stretch statically, always stretch after a run or a good warm-up, not before, so that the muscles are "warm." This improves blood flow to promote the healing that occurs after stretching.

Some studies have shown that a pre-run static stretch session can actually make you run slower, so don't expect your performance on your run to improve if you include static stretching on your speed days, even if it's after a warm-up.

Active Isolated Stretching

With AIS, you release the stretch before the myotatic reflex has a chance to activate, moving only through your natural range of motion and not beyond it. You can stretch on cold muscles before a run or wait until you are done. AIS is pretty relaxing, so I prefer to save it for the end or even another part of the day.

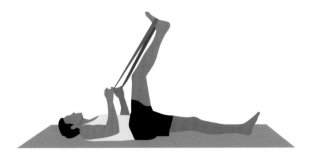

Your main goal with AIS is to work on your mobility. But, as a side effect, you will get more flexible as well. Using this technique, the muscles start to show a greater range of motion by the time you finish each set, and you should be able to reach a little further on the last repeat all without causing damage or pain.

The other feature to AIS is that you are not just using the muscles you are trying to stretch. You enlist the opposing muscle group to bring you into the stretch while allowing the muscle you want to stretch to take a break and relax. A relaxed muscle is more easily stretched than a contracted muscle.

For example, if you want to stretch your hamstrings with AIS, you would lie on your back and lift your leg using the opposing muscles on the front of your leg called the quadriceps. When you use your quads, your hamstrings naturally relax, making them more susceptible to stretching. You stretch the hamstring by lightly pulling the leg back to the point of tightness, never to pain, for two seconds, then release, using your quad to lower the leg instead of just dropping it to the floor. Then you would repeat 8 to 10 times before switching legs.

For many of the stretches done with AIS, a long rope (six to eight feet) is used to help assist you get those last few degrees of motion. For the hamstring, you would put the middle of the rope on the arch of your foot and hold each end in your hands. Lift the leg as far as it naturally goes using only your quads, not the rope, and when you reach the point that you feel a little tight, use the rope to help you reach just a touch farther.

This allows you to reach your full range of motion without having to use a partner, because let's face it, nobody's spouse really wants to help them lift their legs up every day, right?

I've used the hamstrings as an example, but just about every muscle in the body can be stretched using this technique.

The Four Areas Where Flexibility Matters

While, in general, runners don't need to be super flexible, there are four areas of the body where flexibility absolutely counts. The reason for this is improved stride length and efficiency.

There are only two ways to get faster when running: quicken your steps or lengthen your stride. By having a wide range of motion (flexibility) and being able to move well through that range (mobility), you are able to do both.

Hip Extension

Many runners complain that their hips are too tight. They can't get their hips to open up wide and lengthen their stride, or their hips are weak, causing excessive stress lower down the leg, which can lead to knee or IT band issues.

If your hips are so inflexible that your stride can't lengthen out through its full range of motion, you are limiting your speed. And if your hips don't have good enough mobility to move through that range of motion with strength and efficiency, they will quickly get tired. At that point, your brain will be forced to use the weaker muscles in your lower legs to get you down the road, leading to all sorts of disastrous problems for your calves, quads, knees, and hamstrings.

To improve flexibility in your hips, you can use static stretching after you are fully warmed up. The classic runners' stretch, where you open your hips in an exaggerated lunge, is great for this, as is the yoga pose pigeon. But remember, a little goes a long way.

To improve mobility as well as flexibility in the hips, there are a lot of great exercises to try. Lunges in all directions, squats, high knees, step ups, and clams are all good choices.

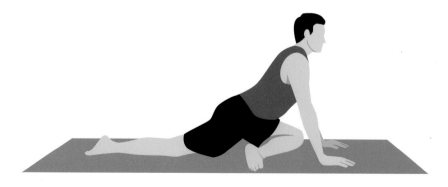

Ankle Extension

The second place a runner needs to be flexible is the ankle. Think about the position your foot is in when it hits the ground. Unless you are a ballerina, your foot will be in the flexed position when it lands. The ability to land on a flexed foot and push off with a pointed foot makes a big impact on how much ground you will cover with each stride. And the joint where that action happens is the ankle.

If you have limited flexibility or mobility in the ankle, your capacity to push off the ground and propel yourself forward will be limited. So it pays to have strong, flexible ankles.

My favorite ankle exercises include a wobble board. If you've never seen one, it's a circle of wood with a center dome on the bottom. You can use it to improve your balance as well as your ankle mobility by practicing flexing and pointing to the front, sides, and back of the board.

You can also work on your ankles just about any time you are sitting down. Work your ankles in all directions, and try holding your point and your flex for several seconds until you feel a good stretch.

Thoracic Spine

This one might not be as obvious. The thoracic spine (t-spine) is the area between the shoulder blades.

Ever watched the end of a marathon? When people are so exhausted that they are running hunched over with their shoulders up to their ears, just shuffling along? If you have limited t-spine mobility, your shoulders will tend to roll forward, your back begins to hunch, and your head will turn into a bowling ball as it extends away from your center of gravity. This happens because you are tired, but this position itself compounds your fatigue since it's so inefficient.

Good mobility in the t-spine also allows for a more efficient arm swing. What your arms do, your legs do, so being able to use your arms well, with very little effort, will make running easier.

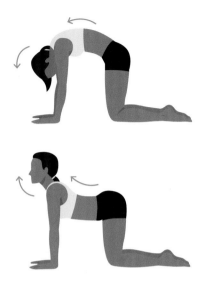

When you run, the arm swings backward, causing a rotation to occur in the t-spine. Meanwhile, the same side leg swings forward. The twist of the spine helps to load the core, which is a good thing. But, if the t-spine is inflexible, the low back takes the load, and that leads to pain and injury.

Good t-spine exercises to try are the yoga moves cat and cow. Start on all fours on the floor and alternate between rounding your back while looking down and arching your back while looking up. Another good one is rolling on a foam roller and allowing your shoulders to drape off the roller and stretch.

The Big Toe

The big toe, or hallux, might be small, but it plays a big role in your running. Hallux mobility and stability are essential to absorb shock, stabilize your stride, store energy, and push off the ground.

Without adequate mobility and strength in your feet and particularly in your big toe, runners can begin to develop all sorts of issues. These include pain in the ankles, shins, knees, hips, and lower back.

To strengthen your feet and big toes, you can perform specific mobility drills while barefoot on either the ground or the grass. Manually stretching your big toes regularly can help as well.

But my favorite way to work my feet is to strength train barefoot. When you take your shoes off and perform challenging strength or balance exercises, your feet are forced to engage as well. Calf raises and lunges in particular require good dorsiflexion of the toes, so you are sneaking in your mobility work at the same time as your strength.

Yes, you need to be a bit more careful not to drop a dumbbell on your foot, but for me, it's worth the slight risk to get my feet stronger without a separate routine.

Simple Balance Training Can Protect You From Running Injuries

Balance is a big buzz word lately. There's work/life balance or balancing marathon training with a hectic schedule. But I want to talk about real physical balance, like being able to stand on one foot with your eyes closed. Excellent balance could be the key to staying injury free.

Why Is Balance Important for Runners?

You may have heard that running is simply a series of hops from one foot to another, so it makes sense that we need to be able to balance on one foot, even if it's for a split second. But I would guess that very few runners actually train their sense of balance, so I'm going to go over why this is important and just how simple this is to do.

Several scientific studies have shown that when a group of athletes trains specifically for better balance, their risk of ankle injuries goes down. One study had the participants use a wobble board for several months and found that two results were at play. The muscles surrounding the ankles got stronger and therefore controlled the ankle in a more stable position, which certainly is what you'd expect from a physical training program that works the ankles.

The second thing the researchers found was that the brain got better at becoming aware of the foot's position relative to the ground and other obstacles. So the brain got stronger at the same time.

This phenomenon of being aware of how your body parts move in relation to your world is called proprioception. And it's extremely important to have a good sense of it to be able to run effortlessly and in control, not to mention avoid injuries AND potholes.

How Balance Helps the Entire Chain

An interesting thing about running injuries is that the place that hurts is rarely the real culprit. More often, injuries result from an imbalance either higher up in the body or lower down the leg.

One example of this is the IT band. The IT band is a long band of connective tissue that runs along the outside of your thigh connecting your pelvis to your knee. It's a common point of irritation and injury in runners and many think that it's from overuse or too much running, too soon. While that definitely can be the cause of IT band issues, the cause could instead be an ankle injury on the opposite leg.

By strengthening the ankle, you are less likely to compensate for an injury with poor form on your good leg, and when you are strengthening your brain's awareness of where your foot is in time and space, you are less likely to twist your ankle in the first place.

How Balance Work Helps Your Stride

What else happens when we train our ankles? We get increased ankle mobility and flexibility, which can help your stride. As I mentioned earlier, runners only need to be flexible (i.e., have a wide range of motion) in four places: the big toe, the ankles, the hips as they extend, and the t-spine. If you have nice, strong, flexible ankles, your push off the ground will be far more efficient.

Simple Balance Exercises

Here are a few quick and easy balance exercises that you can try out. Well, they will be easy once you get the hang of them!

Balance on One Foot

The first thing to do is assess your baseline. Take off your shoes and set a timer for 30 seconds. Raise one knee so your thigh is parallel to the ground, start the timer and close your eyes. Can you stay balanced? It helps to hold your running form while you balance. Activate the glute on the planted foot, keeping your hips tucked underneath you. Keep your shoulders back, and make a 90-degree angle with the elbow opposite the plant foot to mimic a mid-stride stance.

If you fall over before the timer goes off, you have some work to do. Practice a few sets of this every day until you can comfortably balance on each leg for 30 seconds.

Leg Swing

The next exercise is the leg swing. Many runners do leg swings as part of their warm-up routines. Part of it is to improve range of motion in the hips, and the other part of it involves balance and control. Staying in control while you're not on the ground during the swing phase is a key part of efficient form.

Start by standing and holding on to something like a wall or a fence for balance. Stand on one leg and swing the other leg 10 degrees forward and backward, controlling the swinging leg and working up to 30 degrees of swing front to back.

Once you've mastered that, step away from whatever you are holding on to, and do the swings without holding on to anything. Pay attention to your knees, and try to avoid inward and outward rotation during the movement. For even more challenge, swing the opposite arm to meet the swinging leg in its forward position.

Once you become a master at the single leg balance and the no holding on leg swing, it's time to up the ante. Try standing on something wobbly for the single leg stands like a BOSU ball or even a rolled-up yoga mat. Repeat the progression of becoming comfortable with balancing with your eyes closed on an uneven surface for 30 seconds.

Next Level Balance

For an even tougher challenge, add some momentum to your balance drills by bounding on one leg. This is a tough test of functional balance, and it's for athletes whose balance imperfections may not be noticeable until seriously challenged.

Start in a runner's stance, balancing on one leg, and leap onto the opposite leg so that you land in an identical stance. Jump from your left leg onto your right leg, with the left arm swinging, in an exaggerated running hop. When you land, hold the position and stick the landing, like a gymnast at the Olympics. You want knees and torso straight ahead and your pelvis level.

Then you can try bounding front to back, back to front, side to side, and diagonally to maximize your functional balance in all directions.

These exercises don't need to take a lot of time. Five minutes a day or even three times a week is really all you need. Having an excellent sense of balance is not the only thing you need to run your best, but it does play a major role in your ability to progress as a runner, especially if it prevents you from getting injured.

Running Drills

And finally, we have running drills. While often not thought of as a flexibility-improving exercise, running drills are in reality some of the most specific mobility work that runners can perform.

Drills improve functional flexibility even better than static stretching or AIS. They can reinforce the neuromuscular pathways between your brain and legs, which helps them "talk quicker" to each other and helps you become more efficient. Drills also are a form of functional strength training. Not only do they strengthen muscles but they improve the flexibility and mobility of specific joints (like the ankle) needed for powerful, fast running.

Next, they can improve coordination, agility, balance, and proprioception, which is the sense of awareness of where the body is and what it's doing without consciously thinking about it.

And you don't have to wait until your muscles are warm to do drills. They are perfect for warm-ups, cool-downs, rest days, or in the aisles of the grocery store if you like. It's all good!

The only downside to drills is that grown men and women skipping down the street or doing the grapevine look simply ridiculous. But, hey, I think all runners could stand to add just a little bit of silliness to their lives. Don't you agree?

Some classic running drills are butt kicks, high knees, grapevine (also called carioca), bounding, and skipping. In essence, a drill is an exaggerated version of the running movement, so you want to use great form (but exaggerated and extended). Choose a softer surface like grass or a track to lessen the impact you'd get on concrete or asphalt, especially if you are injury prone.

Chapter Seven

Recovery

Recovery is where your body repairs the damage from a workout and makes you stronger.

At the end of a hard workout, your fitness is actually worse than when you began. This is because all that hard effort causes your body to break down muscle fibers, build up lactic acid, and deplete glycogen stores. While it sounds a bit strange that workouts make you worse off when you started, it's pretty obvious that you can't run your fastest 5k 20 minutes after knocking out three miles of hard 400-meter repeats on the track.

Workouts break you down, and recovery builds you up stronger than before.

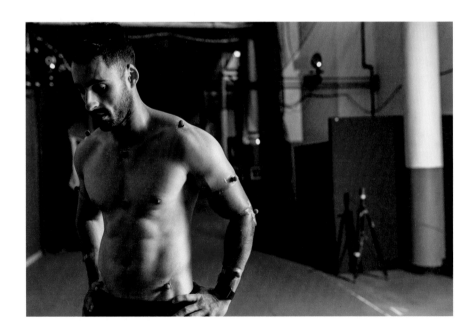

The Science of Soreness: You Don't Need to Be Sore to Be Strong

When you physically work your body a little harder or a little longer than you're used to, it's normal to be sore the next day. Being sore after a long run or lifting weights is a sure sign that you've worked hard and your muscles are growing. And not being sore at the end of a race definitely means that you could have run a lot harder and faster.

Actually, neither one of those statements are true. Soreness is not an indication of a good workout, and lack of soreness is not an indication that you didn't work hard. Seems counterintuitive, but it's true.

So why do we get sore? The truth is that it's not entirely clear why or what the mechanisms involved are, but doing an unfamiliar exercise or one that is prone to soreness or simply being a person that tends to get sore more than others are all factors involved.

Let's say that you head to the gym for the first time in years and grab the biggest dumbbells you can lift. You press and curl and lift and squat and are loving your new fit life, until the next day when even your eyelids hurt to move.

This is called Delayed Onset Muscle Soreness, or DOMS for short. There are a lot of theories of exactly what is happening to cause this pain, but science's best guess is that it relates to inflammation caused by the muscle damage you did in the gym. Inflammation is how your body deals with a lot of problems in the body, and it's essentially like calling out the National Guard to defeat an enemy. Blood rushes into the damaged area to provide nutrients and oxygen for repair, and that extra blood creates heat, swelling, and sometimes pain.

So you are lying in bed, crying in pain, cursing yourself for going too hard in the gym and wondering if you will ever walk again, let alone run.

But soreness doesn't just occur in newbies in January at the gym. It occurs in seasoned athletes and elites as well. There is certainly a kind of twisted masochism in feeling a little sore after an especially brutal trail run or hard intervals at the track. You worked hard, and the soreness is the proof.

Sort of. But what if you could work hard, get the same results, *and* skip the soreness? Sure, you are not getting the same biofeedback loop that rewards you with pain every time you work hard, but imagine walking and, more importantly, running better the next day after a hard workout, with little to no soreness!

Yes, please.

Strength Without Soreness

The key to building muscle and strength without unnecessary soreness is to learn what causes soreness for you and then to learn to train just under that threshold. That could mean strength training more often but with fewer reps or less intensity, or it could mean dialing back the speed on Track Tuesday just a hair so you still run strong but are pain free the next day.

Studies[30] have shown that the sweet spot for optimal muscle growth is just 5 to 10 sets of 10 repetitions for each muscle group per week. That means you can get away with just 10 squats five days a week, and you have your quads and hamstrings covered in less than a minute a day. Fifty squats spread over five to seven days is a lot less likely to produce soreness than fifty squats all at once.

The science backs it up. Studies involving two groups[31] that either did all their strength training on one day or spread it out over five days got the exact same muscle growth at the end of the study, but the five times per week group got it without the soreness.

Eccentric Loads Produce More Soreness

Another factor that tends to produce more soreness is the type of exercise done. Eccentric loads can produce more soreness than concentric movements. But what exactly does that mean?

An eccentric contraction is where the load or stress occurs as the muscle is lengthening, and concentric is the opposite. So imagine a biceps curl. As you curl the dumbbell towards your chest, the biceps shortens. This is concentric. As you lower the weight slowly and lengthen your arm down, that is the eccentric motion (as long as you are doing it slowly and purposefully, instead of just letting gravity pull it down).

Another way to think of eccentric motion is that it's the braking motion. Where do we see the braking motion happen most on a run? If you guessed downhill running, you would be correct. Running downhill eccentrically loads the quads, which is why you might feel soreness the next day if you go flying down a mountain trail.

This is exactly why the Boston Marathon is so challenging even though the net downhill would seem to make it a fast course. The damage that eccentrically loading your quads does in the first half of the race turns your quads into wobbly bowls of jelly by the time you crest Heartbreak Hill.

So does that mean I'm telling you not to run downhill or do eccentric exercises to avoid soreness? Absolutely not. Quite the opposite, in fact. If you are training for Boston or a Revel race with lots of downhill, you absolutely need eccentric training, and all runners can benefit from it. But a little goes a long way, and spreading out your strength training and your downhill running over days or even weeks can get you stronger and more durable without the pain.

Gain Without the Pain

Okay, so let's say you are all jazzed up about this and vow to never be sore again. You try all these tips and still end up sore. What gives? Well, you could be someone who is just naturally more prone to feeling sore. You can try cutting back the weight and intensity a little and see if that helps, and it certainly should help some. But for some people, a little soreness will still happen at times, and it doesn't mean that anything is necessarily wrong.

Lack of Soreness

And finally, what if you are the opposite and you don't feel sore? Does that mean that you could have gone faster? This is a very common experience, especially in runners as they grow and improve. The week after your first marathon was a miserable suffer fest where you couldn't even look at a set of stairs without wincing. But your next one, even though you ran it faster, wasn't quite as bad. And then the next was even better and so on until finally you got that marathon dream PR you'd always been hoping for, and you hardly even felt it the next day. Could you have gone faster?

Maybe you could have, but your lack of muscle soreness has nothing to do with it. Biopsies of experienced marathon runner's legs still show markedly high levels of muscle damage regardless of whether they report being sore or not.

Most likely the reason you are not sore is that your body has adapted to the stimulus of running long and hard and no longer calls out the National Guard with pain sirens blaring quite as loud. The bottom line is that soreness is a poor indicator of anything useful for your training and can be avoided for most runners most of the time.

You can still run hard, lift hard, and become a fitter and faster runner (while still being able to walk normally). The trick is to sneak up on your fitness by doing a little consistent work every day (rather than killing yourself).

Now let's take a look at what you can do after a good workout or run to help you maximize the benefits of all the work you did.

Refuel and Rehydrate

The first step of recovery is eating and drinking. Even on a cool day, you lose fluid through sweat when you are working hard, so grab some water after every run. Clearly, on hot days and after harder workouts, you'll need to replace more lost fluid, but don't be ridiculous here. Your body is smart, so drinking to thirst after running is usually all you need.

If you are not a particularly thirsty runner, you can get most of your water needs met if you include lots of water-rich foods in your diet like fruits and vegetables, which, of course, also provide all sorts of other great benefits. But topping off with water after a run is always a good idea.

Chapter three goes into more detail about recovery foods, and for the most part, the best plan is to just keep it simple! If you just ran a workout that beat you up a bit, whether that's from intensity or distance, then making good food choices right after your run is more important. If you just ran an easy or short run, whatever that means to you, you should not be depleted, so you can either wait until your next meal to eat or you can just have something light.

As always, whole, unprocessed, real food primarily or entirely from plants is your best bet in running and in life and will enhance your recovery.

But don't stress out too much about the exact timing of your nutrition. Your body is smart, and it will use the nutrients you feed it, whenever they are available. Unless you are a highly competitive runner who is working out twice a day, you really don't need to focus on perfect timing of eating after runs.

Mobility, Stretching, Massage

Okay, so you ran hard and had something to drink and something to eat. What's next? This can be a great time to squeeze in a little preventative maintenance like stretching or mobility work.

Stretching, and specifically AIS, not only feels great after a tough run (after all, you get to lie down!), but it can help increase mobility and range of motion. This makes your running more efficient with less effort, which is something we all want. (More on this in chapter six.)

Other things you can do to help yourself recover include foam rolling, heat, and massage. If you are lucky enough to have access to a hot tub or a massage therapist, those are great tools. But, if not, a foam roller and a warm compress or hot bath are really all you need!

Sleep Your Way to Better Running

And last, but certainly not least, is sleep. Sleep is absolutely critical to the repair process. High level athletes can sleep 9 to 10 hours a day. You might not be able to get that much, but if you are waking up tired and are wondering why your workouts aren't going well, lack of good sleep is likely a major culprit.

I have battled insomnia on and off for as long as I can remember, and I'm literally so tired of it that I've been learning all that I can so that I can sleep deeper and wake up refreshed.

One thing I've noticed personally is that when I'm running more, I sleep better. When I was logging lots and lots of miles, I had no trouble conking out for eight or nine hours a night, so perhaps more running is part of my solution.

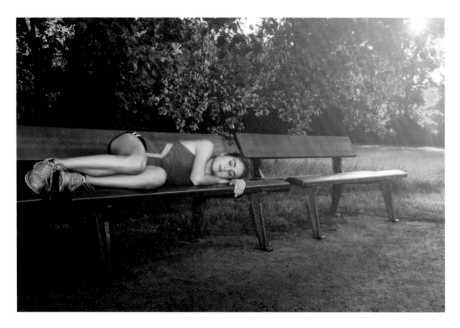

Lack of Sleep Affects Everything

We all know that sleep is important, but most of us in our high-stress society shortchange ourselves by choice. We wake up at four a.m. to run, because that is the only time that there is no demand on our time from our family or from work. But unless we turn out the lights at eight p.m. the night before, we end up being chronically sleep deprived, which causes a laundry list of problems for our health, well-being, longevity, and running performance.

Chronic sleep deprivation, which can be as slight as only getting seven hours of sleep a night instead of eight, will not only make you tired, but it reduces your motor skills, endurance, and time to exhaustion, impairs your cardiovascular, metabolic, and respiratory capabilities, increases your risk of injury, and decreases your ability to cool yourself through sweating. Obviously, these are all things that we are looking to improve through training, and we might be unknowingly sabotaging our efforts every night!

Injury Risk and Repair

A 2014 study[32] of youth athletes found that chronic lack of sleep is associated with increased sports injuries in adolescent athletes. The researchers looked at a lot of differing factors, and hours of sleep was a better predictor of injury than even hours spent practicing. Now, I would guess that most of you reading this aren't student athletes, and this is an area that certainly needs more study, but it would make sense that the same would hold true for adults as well.

If you are already injured, getting enough sleep can help you heal and recover more quickly, and not getting enough can slow the whole process down. When you are asleep, your brain and your body are actually highly active. As you fall into the deeper stages of sleep, blood flow increases to your muscles, which brings oxygen and nutrients that help muscles recover and repair and damaged cells regenerate.

Your pituitary gland is also wide awake as you sleep. When the body enters the sleep stage known as non-REM sleep, the pituitary gland releases growth hormones that stimulate muscle repair and growth. If you are not getting enough sleep, you're not getting enough growth hormone, which will make it harder for your body to recover from injuries.

Inflammation and the Immune System

Another hormone that is released while you sleep is prolactin, which helps regulate inflammation. Again, the fewer hours you sleep, the less this helpful hormone is released, which makes you more susceptible to inflammation in the body. Chronic inflammation not only makes injury recovery more difficult, but it also puts you at risk of another injury, starting the cycle all over again.

Short sleeping also suppresses your immune system, making your vulnerable to illness. Studies have shown that individuals who slept less than seven hours a night were nearly three times as likely to develop an infection compared with those who slept eight hours or more.

Sleep and Performance

Now, let's talk about performance. Science has not been able to figure out all of the direct mechanisms of the relationship of sleep and performance, but multiple studies have shown a definite link.

When it comes to endurance performance, most research has demonstrated that sleep deprivation inhibits performance, and the most obvious indicator is an increase in perceived exertion. Clearly, when you feel tired, everything feels harder, and you want to stop sooner. Those negative voices inside your head are a lot harder to fight when you are simply fighting to stay awake.

Recovery between your runs is also affected by less-than-ideal sleeping. A study on cyclists found that after just one night of inadequate sleep, the subjects performed four percent worse on a time trial the next day, perhaps suggesting that restricted sleep impaired their recovery between workouts.

Another effect of sleep loss is that your body won't have enough time to adequately stock up on glycogen, the fuel required to run fast. Pre-exercise muscle glycogen stores have been found to be decreased after sleep deprivation, which means the dreaded bonk comes a lot sooner on race day.

There is still a lot of research to be done on the role of sleep, but study after study makes it clear that regular, quality sleep makes absolutely everything better. Athletes probably need more sleep than non-athletes, but the exact amount has yet to be quantified by science.

Chronic vs. Acute Lack of Sleep

One poor night of sleep (e.g., tossing and turning with nerves before race day) has not been proven to do much harm with regard to your race performance, assuming you have tapered and recovered well. But chronic sleep loss night after night, even by just an hour or so, had been associated with major negative effects on both health and performance.

Ways to Improve Your Sleep

So how do you get more of the good stuff? The first step, which you've already done, is to learn the importance of sleep and prioritize it. Sleep is not just part of a healthy lifestyle, it is the foundation of health, which is why we spend a third of our lives in bed.

Here are some tips from the National Institutes of Health[33]:

1. Keep a regular sleep schedule, and go to bed at the same time every night. You can't make up for lost sleep on the weekends. It just doesn't work that way.
2. Exercise in the morning, hopefully with lots of sunshine, or early afternoon to set your circadian rhythm. If evening is the only time you have to run, schedule it at least two or three hours before bed.
3. Avoid caffeine seven to eight hours before bed.
4. Avoid alcohol two to three hours before sleeping.

5.   Avoid large meals late at night. A small snack is okay, but a full belly makes it harder to sleep.
6.   Don't take naps after three p.m.
7.   Relax before bed with reading, music, or a hot bath.
8.   Keep your bedroom dark, quiet, and cool. If yours isn't, use a sleep mask and ear plugs. (This especially has made a difference for me!)
9.   Keep the electronics out of the bedroom, and avoid their blue light within a couple hours of bedtime.
10. Don't let stressing about lack of sleep cause you not to sleep! (This is a big one for me!) If you are lying awake in bed for more than 20 minutes, get up and go to another room and read a book until you are sleepy.

While there is still a lot of research to be done on sleep, it is abundantly clear that athletes and everybody else need to make sleep a top priority for top health and performance.

Recovery Changes as You Age

Alright, let's say you do all of those things I mentioned, and you wake up the next day after a great night of shuteye. The vast majority of people, especially as we age, are not sufficiently recovered enough the next day to run well. Younger runners can process the damage more efficiently and, in general, have quicker recovery times, but even the fittest athletes in the world recognize that back-to-back hard running can only happen for so long before they dig a hole they can't get out of.

That's why recovery days, whether it's true rest or just easy running, are essential. If you are running easy the day after a workout, make sure it truly is easy enough to feel restorative. If you run too fast on an easy day, which most beginner runners and even some experienced runners do, you are simply pushing your recovery farther into the future. A medium-paced run is not restorative, even if you think you are running easy. Easy needs to feel slow!

If you are struggling in your workouts, the number one reason is because you are not recovering well enough, so take those easy days easy enough that you feel fresh and fast on your hard days and slow as molasses on your easy days.

Like most things running, your recovery needs will change as you age, so that perfect recovery plan that you worked so hard to figure out will eventually have to be altered to meet your changing needs as a mature athlete, so don't get too locked in, and always be willing to reevaluate.

Younger runners might find that they can bounce back from a hard Tuesday track session ready to smash a Thursday tempo run and then crush a Saturday long run. But don't be surprised that you find that what worked for you at 25 doesn't work for you at 45. (Are you surprised? Of course not!)

You can be in the best shape of your life in your 40s, 50s, and beyond, but that doesn't mean you can recover like a 20-year-old. You might find that, after your Tuesday track day, tempos feel much better on Fridays instead of Thursdays, pushing your long run to Sunday.

The majority of athletes I coach are over the age of 40, and I often encourage masters athletes to build in two recovery days between hard sessions. This doesn't mean you are working any less hard than the young guns from the running shop. It means you are working smarter for your individual needs.

The Second Speed Day Is Optional

The next thing I encourage my athletes to do is to consider the second workout of the week as optional. So if you really tore it up at the track, consider letting that be your hard day of the week, and don't run the hard tempo this week. This will save your legs for a better long run that weekend, leaving you stronger instead of more broken down.

And if you are really feeling that runner's anxiety of not working hard enough, add a few strides (see chapter two) to the end of your easy run on the day you would have had the second workout. That way, you are staying in touch with your speed, but you are not running so hard that you need more recovery.

With proper recovery, you are not going to feel exhausted all the time, and your hard days will get faster and better and so will your races. And I'd be willing to bet you're going to feel better and be nicer to be around. So if you don't want to recover better for yourself, please do it for the rest of us!

Chapter Eight

Mindset

Learn to train your mind to be as strong as your body

Running Is a Practice, Not a Test

As a coach, I've worked with hundreds of athletes, and it's remarkable how some runners really get themselves tied up in knots over their splits, their workouts, and their races. Yet other runners seem to just go with the flow, embracing what comes, both good and bad.

Sure, everyone gets disappointed when something doesn't go as expected, in both life and in running, but it's fascinating how some athletes will spin a bad run into a lesson for the future, while others spin into a downward spiral of self-loathing.

It's more than just having a positive attitude versus a negative one. It's a completely different outlook. Let me take you behind the curtain a little to see what we see as coaches.

When I'm creating workouts for athletes, I'm trying to create a certain type of stimulation at a certain time in the cycle to elicit a certain type of growth in the athlete. This could be focusing on the aerobic system or the anaerobic system or

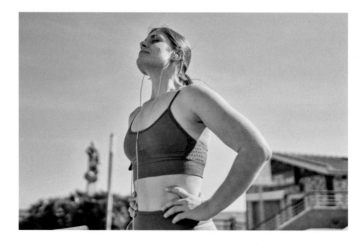

perhaps building stamina or raw speed—whatever makes sense for the particular phase in the cycle or the day of the week. The way I choose those paces is to extrapolate from recent race results or recent workouts using formulas, calculators, or estimators or just taking an educated guess based on what I know about the athlete.

In other words, I make up your paces for you. They are not handed down on a tablet from God, written in stone. They are created with the intent of getting you to a certain level of effort to get the desired response. They also assume that you are running in perfectly cool weather, with no wind, on a dead-flat course, with the stars aligned to your zodiac sign.

So when you miss your assigned paces by a second on a hot and humid day, you are really missing a fairly arbitrary time goal. You can either blame yourself for not being good enough, or you can choose to look at the larger picture. If your effort was there, the purpose was achieved, whether it was off by a few seconds or not.

The written assignment your coach gave you is not as simple as run x distance at x pace and repeat; it is far more nuanced than that. So instead of just focusing on the numbers, learn the purpose of the workout and aim for the spirit intended, whether or not the paces line up.

Purpose-Based Running

Some runners have a really hard time with the concept of purpose-based running and are generally inflexible when it comes to numbers on the watch (well, let's face it, runners are generally inflexible in a lot of places; for more, see chapter six).

I get it. The numbers are important. They are a measure of how we are doing and if we are getting better or worse.

One of the beautiful things about running is that it is seemingly so simple. Put on your shoes and try to run farther or faster or both farther and faster than before. But, to many runners, when you don't run faster one day, something is wrong. You've failed.

So you try harder, run more distance, run more often, and run more intensely. That will work for a while (until it doesn't) and you end up breaking something, physically, mentally, or both.

It's challenging to let go of the numbers and use effort. People get really worked up about this idea, too, probably more so than when coaches give them exact paces. What does a hard effort mean? How slow is easy effort? When you say run hard up the hill for 30 seconds, how fast is that?

This response is completely valid and understandable. As an athlete, I want to know if I'm getting better and moving towards my goal, so if the coach just says run medium hard, how do I know if I'm too medium or too hard? Sure, the more you run, the more familiar you will be with what that feels like, but it sure feels unsettling to not "know" if you are succeeding or failing.

And let's be clear. I'm not saying don't use your watch. Use it as the tool it is. But temper it with how the workout felt in the conditions you were given. Understand the purpose behind the paces.

Because your workout is not a test. It's a brick that you lay every day to build a house. If you went out there on a hard day and ran hard, that's one brick. If you went out on your easy day and really ran easy, that's a brick. If you rested on your rest day, that's another brick. You don't test the foundation of your house with every third brick you lay or you would weaken the house. Your fitness is the same way.

It can help to think of your running as a whole instead of labeling each run as good or bad or something in between. Every day that you run, you become a better runner. You are practicing your craft every time you lace up, no matter what the results are.

You Can't Fail at Practice

When you judge your running by the numbers on a clock, there is a clear "pass/fail" trap that's easy to fall into. You either ran x, or you failed.

But when you instead shift your focus to running as a practice for better running in the future, even "failed" runs are a success.

Other activities lend themselves to this approach very easily. Take yoga, for example. We say that we are "practicing" yoga when we hit the mat, and every time we have a session, we become better at it. There are no numbers in yoga, so there's not always a clear way to tell us if we were "good" or "bad" that day. But maybe your heels got a little bit closer to the floor in downward facing dog one day, or maybe you were able to hold triangle pose just a few breaths longer than before. These are non-numerical signs of progress, and the only way to achieve them is with steady and consistent practice.

Running can be just like that. Especially as we age and those magic numbers get harder and harder to reach.

On easy days, think about how jogging is the very best form of practice for running and racing faster. On hard days, think about how you are choosing to push yourself through discomfort to become a more fluid and efficient runner who can handle the high stress of running hard without letting negative thoughts overwhelm you and slow you down. And on your rest days, delight in the thought that your body is absorbing all the hard work you've put in and is building a stronger version of yourself, confident in the knowledge that good rest makes you better, not weaker.

Because the best runners are not the ones that punish themselves day after day. They are the ones that build a consistent running practice, learn from their mistakes, and see every day as a small building block of a very large structure.

And you can have this, too. It just takes practice.

Mastering Your Mind When You Want to Quit

Most of the runners I coach want to know how to build mental toughness. When things get hard in a race or tough workout, they tend to break down, slow down, or give up. They might feel like they have the physical fitness to complete the workout well but feel like something is holding them back mentally.

You Can Train Your Brain

Before I get into this, everything that I will talk about here has to do with effort-based pain. I'm not trying to teach you how to run though a pulled hamstring or a stress fracture. This is all about getting the best out of yourself when the effort gets high, not pushing through injuries. So with that out of the way, let's get into your brain, shall we?

Your Dueling Selves

When we run, there is often an internal struggle going on between the desire to push and the desire to stop. Your brain is very protective of the body and relies on you not killing yourself when you run. So if the brain gets any hint that you are doing something out of the ordinary, it will sound the alarm, beginning with negative thought patterns.

"This hurts," a little voice will say. "I'm breathing too hard, this is too fast, I can't do this," and on and on and on.

The simple way to beat this is by training so well and so carefully that you always run within your ability, which gets better and better with time and practice, and never trigger a sense of panic from the brain. You practice running hard so when it's time to run hard, your brain is used to it. But c'mon, we race to push ourselves! We want to know how fast we can get from point A to point B, and if we stick with what the brain is happy with, we will never reach our true potential.

If you are going to push, you will get push back from your brain. So, how do you deal with it?

Don't Skip the Warm-Up

Physically, besides good training, making sure you are warmed up can make a huge difference. If you hit the starting line cold and fly out of the gates, your body thinks you are being chased by a saber-toothed tiger and will flood you with adrenaline. That's a good thing since it will help you run faster, but when the rush is over, the shocked brain will be ready to calm down and slow down.

But if you ease into your speed with a good warm-up and a conservative start, the brain gets a heads up, if you will, and says, "Oh yeah, we're running now. I've done this before." And the chance of the panicked negative talk lessens or at least gets pushed down the road.

Anticipate the Arrival of Negative Thoughts

Being prepared mentally for the battle ahead is just as important as being physically ready, and some say it's even more important. The first step is to expect that it's coming. You should not be surprised that your brain wants to stop you from doing hard things, and thoughts will arise that will tell you to stop, slow down, take a break.

Give Your Negative Voice A Name

By creating an identity for your negative self-talk, you are, in a sense, externalizing it, which helps you separate the temporary emotion from what you really want. It's not really "you" who wants to quit; it's an uninvited guest in your head.

For me this voice was always very sweet and kind, disguising her true evil. She is Nancy, a sweet Southern granny, who just wants me to slow down and eat some cupcakes with her. "You're tired, dear. Why don't you slow down?" she says. "No one will be upset with you if you slow down, sweetie. Your family will still love you if you quit. Why are you doing this anyway?" she asks.

It's hard to argue with Nancy, because she's right! I am tired, and my family will still love me if I don't run my goal time. And when you are tired and still running, it's hard to come up with a good argument against such sound logic.

So the trick is to prepare ahead of time. I know Nancy is coming along for the ride, but she doesn't get to drive the bus. She is sweet, but overprotective. She is kind, but honestly, she's getting in my way.

Creating an identity for my negative voice helps me separate it from myself and my true goals and dreams, even though of course it is a part of myself. If I make Nancy just another obstacle in the journey, rather than letting her get a say in the decision making, then it's easier to say, "Shut up, Nancy!" and keep on running.

Feelings Aren't Facts

My next tip is to remember that feelings aren't facts. You can even use that as a mantra when things get hard in a race and say it over and over again to yourself. Feelings aren't facts. Your brain creates feelings, and they are as ephemeral as the clouds on a summer day. Feelings are real, and I'm not saying you are imagining them, but they are creations based on past experience and what your brain is concluding based on perceptions of the facts around you.

So when you are running hard, your brain might say, "This is hard." And when you say that, you might think, "Hey, I'm right, this really is hard." And then, "Yes, this does feel hard, and now it feels even harder." And on and on the circle of brain chatter goes, a spiral of self-fulfilling prophecy.

But if, instead, when you think, "This is hard," you answer, "Yes, but things will change, just hang on," you're acknowledging that while racing is certainly difficult, every fleeting emotion can and will pass.

Arguing, both in running and in life, is exhausting, and I want to use that energy for speed, not a brain battle.

Take The Words Away

If the arguing gets too intense, take the vocabulary away. Instead of allowing your brain to think whole thoughts, reduce your thoughts to numbers and start counting. This tip really works and lots of runners use it to drown out their noisy brains.

I prefer to simply count to ten over and over again, and the reason I don't go higher is because the rhythms of the lower numbers are easier to time with my steps. "One, two, three" is easier to run to than "twenty-five, twenty-six, twenty-seven," for example.

Counting provides a distraction from all the hard work you are doing and helps you forget for a few moments that you are running hard because you are not focused on everything that hurts. The chatter is limited to a task you learned before kindergarten, so it's deeply familiar to your agitated brain.

Hyper-Focusing Can Help

On the flip side of distraction is hyper-focus, and that can be equally effective in keeping your head in the game. Many runners like to do a head-to-toe form check when things get tough. In one sense, this is paradoxically still a distraction technique since focusing on keeping your head up and your shoulders down and back can help distract you from your screaming quads, but for most people who like this technique, it doesn't feel like a distraction. The attention you are paying to your form physically helps you run more efficiently, which means that running hard is less effortful.

Get Out of Your Head and Look Around

My next tip is, if things are getting too intense inside of your head, get out of it!

Look around and start playing some mental games with the things and people around you. Maybe it's picking out a telephone pole and just trying to run your best

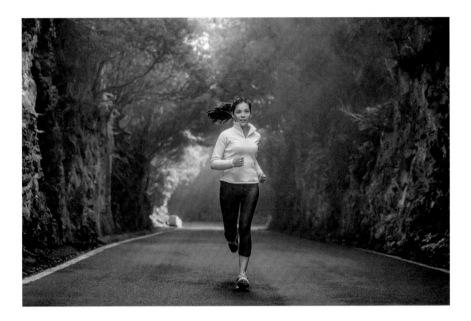

until that point. Maybe it's seeing the guy in the red hat in front of you and seeing if you can reel him in like a fish and catch him. Or maybe it's breaking into a smile (which is a natural pain killer, by the way) and giving that little kid on the side of the road a high five.

Running and racing well does not have to be all about biting the bullet and grimacing your way to the finish line. In fact, relaxing your face eases tension and makes running easier. If you tend to get too tense about things mentally, you are very likely also getting tense physically, which costs precious energy that should be going to your legs. If that's you, think "relaxed fast, relaxed fast" or something similar as your mantra.

Racing your best often involves pushing beyond what you've been trained to do physically. But, if you practice some mental coping strategies during your hard days of training, you will be far more prepared for the huge mental challenge on race day.

Mantras

The word "mantra" is Sanskrit and means "instrument for thinking." It's a mental tool that you use to create a way of thinking that positively enhances your running performance. They are short, positive phrases that you repeat to yourself in your head that can help shift your focus to what you want to be thinking instead of what you really are thinking, which when racing can be anything but positive.

Mantras have been used for centuries to focus the mind in meditation, and you can use them while running to help shift the inevitable negative thoughts into positive self-talk.

Running is hard and even painful at times. When you are racing from point A to point B, there will be times when your legs burn, you get a side stitch, you become out of breath, or you feel like you are overheating. You start to think, "Why am I doing this again? This is hard!" There is a huge part of you that just wants to stop the madness and relax. But then there's this other part of you that loves the thrill of racing well, and despite what you have to go through to get there, that part of you wants to get to the finish line in the shortest possible amount of time.

So how do you quiet the devil on your shoulder and turn up the volume on the angel? Mantras can help boost the positive voice that you want to hear.

Unique to You

The first thing to know about good mantras is that they have to be uniquely inspiring to you. Borrowing someone else's mantra will only work if you are personally connected to that phrase.

When coming up with a good mantra, think of the times in a race or a hard workout where you struggled and the negative talk got the best of you. If you could have a do over that day, how would you rewrite the words in your head?

For example, let's say that you got to a point in the race when you know you needed to turn the effort up but felt like you couldn't. In your head, you were probably thinking something like, "I can't do this. I'm slowing down. I can't, I can't, I can't." When those thoughts cross your mind and you begin to repeat them over and over again, it reinforces the effort and discomfort you are feeling. In fact, whatever you repeat to yourself over and over again in your head becomes reinforced, so you really want to make it positive!

A good mantra shifts the thoughts that compound the pain you're feeling to thoughts that help you transcend it. In other words, what you think is what you feel. But, you have to truly believe it, or it doesn't really work.

Short, Positive, Easy to Remember

A good mantra needs to be short, positive, and easy to remember. Your brain will be too tired to recite Shakespeare in a marathon, so make sure that you limit it to a few words. You'll also want to come up with several of them that you can pull out as needed during various points in the race. If you are struggling to come up with some on your own, allow me to share a few of mine.

One of my frustrations while racing was not running to the potential I knew I had trained for. When I got to a stretch of the race where things got tough, the negative side of my brain gave me plenty of excuses to use to slow down. So when I got to the finish time slower than I had hoped, I felt upset with myself for letting my foot off the gas. I wanted to be proud of the effort I put out, no matter what the clock said. So one of my mantras became, "Make yourself proud." And it worked.

Another one I've used in a marathon is simply, "this mile." My thoughts in the early part of the race would inevitably be something along the lines of, "My God, I can't believe how far I have to go. If I'm feeling like this now, how am I going to make it 26.2 miles?" Or if one of my mile splits came in slow, I would begin to think the worst and be tempted to give up. To combat those thoughts, I knew I needed to stay present and shift my focus to the mile that I was running at the moment. I needed to forget about the past miles and not worry about the future miles. The words "this mile" helped me do just that.

Mantras for Specific Challenges

When it comes to mantras, more is better. A good practice is to think of all the situations where you typically struggle on a run and come up with a positive mantra to counteract them.

One common experience when running a long race or workout is to lose your focus somewhere in the middle. Your mind might not be necessarily negative, but you glance at your watch and realize that you've let your mind wander and you've fallen off pace. This would happen to me, and I ended up stealing a quote that one of my kids' teachers would say to get the class to pay attention. It was "Hocus pocus, everybody focus." The silliness of that one would make me smile, which is a natural painkiller, and it would remind me to get my head back in the game.

Some people use mantras that help them remember good form or get up hills quickly. If hills have been an issue for you in the past, you might try to flip that into a positive. You could try, "I own this hill," or "I'm smooth on hills," or "recover at the top." To help you keep good form, I like repeating "relaxed fast," which inspires me to relax my face and my shoulders to save energy for my legs.

When my legs start to complain that they are working too hard, instead of telling myself that my legs are tired, I say my legs feel alive!

When the wind smacks me in the face and running feels way harder than it should, I imagine the force of the wind helping to fill my lungs with oxygen, so I say to myself, "more oxygen."

You Have to Believe to Achieve

Now, you might be listening to the words that I use and think they are silly or that you'd never believe it if you said them to yourself. And that's because there is no universal mantra that works for everyone. You need to believe it for it to work. And just like a new pair of shoes or a new sports bra, you don't want to try a new mantra out for the first time on race day.

So come up with a few that you think might work for you, and try them out in training. Maybe you need to write them on the back of your hand with a marker to remember them, but test them out over and over again so that on race day they become second nature.

The mind is incredibly powerful, and what you think while you race can work for you or against you. With a little practice, you can create an effective mental tool that can help you get the very best out of yourself and make yourself proud.

If you'd like to dive deeper into developing a stronger mindset for running, you can find mental strength training courses at theplantedrunner.com.

Chapter Nine

Ready to Race

Learn the different types of runs and workouts that will prepare you for a goal race

Race Day Rules: Tips for Racing Your Best

If you've never raced before and are just getting started, you might not know what to expect on race day. Not just from a performance point of view but what the whole race experience will be like.

Racing is fun and exciting, and it will go a lot better if you do a little planning and understand the rules. So let's get into a few dos and don'ts for your next race.

Race Rule #1: No Cheating!

This seems too obvious to even bring up, but you might be surprised how many well-meaning runners find themselves on the wrong side of the rules.

Cutting the course, using someone else's bib, accepting payment to run for someone else, selling bibs, making fake bibs, using performance enhancing drugs, or whatever else that could constitute not running fair and square is not cool. You are not only cheating yourself, but you are cheating every single runner out there who is not cheating. And in the case of races that require qualification, like the Boston Marathon, cheating to get into the race steals a spot from someone who didn't cheat. Earn your spot or go do something else.

Race Rule #2: Learn the Logistics

Before the race begins, learn as much as you can about the logistics of the particular race you've entered. That means read the website, read the emails, ask questions at the expo (if there is one), and generally figure out where you are supposed to be and when. If you have family or friends cheering you on, make sure you all know where the best place to meet up is at the end of the race. It can often be quite crowded at the end of big events, so designate this ahead of time.

Some small races offer same-day registration. That might seem like a convenient option if you are on the fence about the race, but it rarely is for both you or the race organizers. Pre-register so you can show up prepared and avoid the long lines and the organizers can plan properly.

Race Rule #3: Arrive Early

This is one instance in life where being on time is actually horribly late. You want to be sure that you have enough time to check in, get your bib, warm up, and use the porta potty at least once, maybe even twice. Big, major races have long lines, and the last thing you want is to be in line when the gun is about to go off (believe me, I've been there!). And while you are there, please do your very best to keep it clean. Enough said.

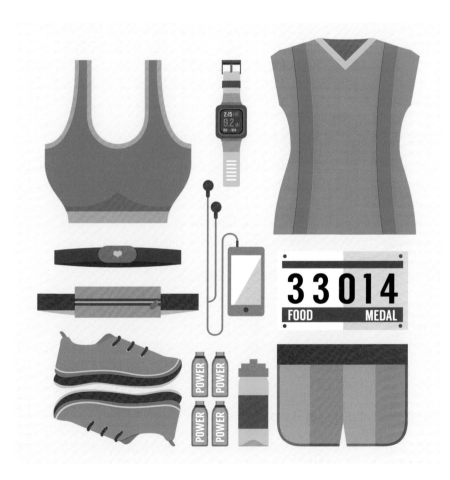

Race Rule #4: Bibs Go in Front

Make sure you pin your bib on the front of you. It could be your shirt or your shorts, but make sure it's on the front. The obvious benefit is being able to find yourself in your race photos, but it's also to help race staff know who you are and that you deserve to be there.

I bring this up because some runners find that a bib on their chest gets in the way or is a distraction. So they pin it on their back or down their leg or some other strange spot. Bibs are an important part of the sport, so keep it front and center!

Race Rule #5: Line Up According to Predicted Finish Time

On the starting line, line up according to how fast you are. That means fastest in the front and walkers in the back. Major races have seeded corrals, and volunteers ensure that everyone is in the right order when they line up, but help them out by staying where you should be. If you are running with a faster friend, you should line up at the slower pace, not the faster pace. This allows the congestion to clear as quickly as possible so that faster runners are not forced to zig and zag around slower ones.

Race Rule #6: Be Smart About Headphones

Running and racing with music can be fun and a great motivator. But, while waiting for the gun to go off, turn your headphones down or off or at least take one earbud out so that you can hear any last-minute instructions from the race officials. And remember that some races do not allow headphones, and most don't allow them for prize winners, so that is something you should be sure to look into ahead of time.

Race Rule #7: Only Two Across, Please

Once the race begins, excited runners will be jostling for space, determined to get that PR. So if you are there as a fun run and plan to gab with five of your running buddies while taking up half the race course, please don't. Two across is fine, but more than that, and you turn the race into an obstacle course for the rest of the field.

Race Rule #8: Polite Passing

If you'd like to pass someone and it's crowded, let them know with a polite "on your left" or "on your right." If they are wearing headphones and don't seem to hear you, it's okay to give them a gentle touch on the elbow to let them know. If you are the one being passed, don't be that guy blocking the person who wants to get by. Shift over a bit and smile because you know that you will probably catch that runner later because you have wisely chosen not to go out too fast.

Race Rule #9: Be Good With the Gross

As you are running, you might feel the need to do something that would definitely not be considered polite in the real world but is perfectly normal in racing. So if you have to spit, consider the wind direction, and aim to avoid other runners. If you need to get rid of other bodily fluids and can't get to a port a potty in time, do your best to get off the course and be discreet as you can.

If you have to stop for any reason—to tie your shoe, to take a break, or to answer your phone (yes, people really do this)—please move to the side and step off the course.

Race Rule #10: Pay Attention!

Some big courses are completely closed off to traffic but others are not, so pay attention to your surroundings and the instructions of volunteers, because it still your job to avoid getting run over by an unsuspecting car.

Race Rule #11: Share the Lead When Drafting

On windy days, it can be very helpful to draft behind other runners to let them block the wind for you. In crowded races, this is fairly easy to do without being annoying to the runner ahead of you, as long as you keep a few feet of distance and aren't clipping their heels. But in a sparse race, it can feel downright spooky to have someone ghosting you the whole race. So the key is to communicate and share the burden. If you are drafting for a while, summon some energy to take the lead, and take turns. Working together can help you both have a better race than both of you fighting the wind alone.

Race Rule #12: Aid Station Etiquette

Alright, so you've been running for a mile or two and come up to your first aid station. These can flow smoothly and seamlessly, or they can be hazardous clusters. If the aid station is on the right, ease to the right to grab a cup with your right hand instead of darting suddenly in front of others. Keep moving as you grab your cup.

If you plan to stop, move past the table and then stop; don't stop right in front of the volunteers because this blocks other people's access.

Once you are done with your cup, you get extra points if you can shoot it directly into a garbage can, but if not, getting it as close as possible to an aid station is the next best thing. And don't be that runner that tosses a half-full cup over your shoulder, showering the guy behind you. Bring the cup down to waist level and toss it from there.

Race Rule #13: Thank the Volunteers

Oh, and don't forget to thank the volunteers while you are there! They are probably spending a lot more time on the course than you are, making sure that thousands of people have a great race, so a quick thank you goes a very long way. Not to mention, simply the act of smiling lowers your perception of effort, so that "thank you" you give is not only good manners but is good racing!

Race Rule #14: Enjoy the Celebration!

When you get to the finish line, be sure to cross both sets of timing mats with a smile on your face so you look good in the race photo, and then stop your watch.

Big races often have long finishing chutes, so take out your headphones so you can hear the instructions of the volunteers, and keep moving. Enjoy the post-race snacks, and move through the chute to meet up with your family and friends at your pre-designated meeting area.

The awards ceremony can be a great way to celebrate the event, mingle with the winners, or pick up some hardware for yourself, so be sure to stick around for that if you can and celebrate everyone's accomplishment.

Racing can be a fun and rewarding experience, but it's certainly made better if everyone is on the same page with what to expect.

Race Your First or Best 5k

One of the most popular race distances out there for recreational and professional runners alike is the 5k. A 5k race is 3.1 miles long, and if you live in any decently-sized town or city in the United States, you could find a 5k race just about every weekend, especially in the nice-weather months.

Part of the reason they are so popular is because they are so accessible. Most people can walk three miles, and most relatively fit people can run 3 miles, so the 5k is a fund raiser's dream race distance. If you are just starting to get in shape, a 5k is an admirable and achievable goal and a great way to showcase your newfound fitness.

More seasoned runners show up at 5k races to test their skills, polish up their speed, or to get a hard workout in with thousands of their closest friends in the middle of their marathon training. The beauty of a 5k for these runners is that it's long enough to still be highly aerobic but short enough to really crank down some speed. And unlike a marathon, racing a 5k won't leave you walking funny for the next several days, meaning you can slip in 5ks almost as much as you like in a marathon buildup without missing a beat of training with extra recovery days.

What's a "Fast" 5K?

The 5k, or 5000 meter, race has been around since at least 1897. As of this writing, the men's world record, held by Ugandan Joshua Cheptegei, is 12:35, and the women's world record is 14:29, run by Ethiopian Senbere Teferi. It's doubtful that any of the tape breakers at your local Turkey Trot will come anywhere close to these blisteringly fast paces, but it's fun to dream, isn't it?

So What's Considered "Fast" for a 5k for a Mere Mortal?

Well, if you are walking a 5k, it would take you somewhere around 45 to 60 minutes to complete. Most recreational runners would be pretty happy with a 25-minute 5k or less, which is 5 minutes per kilometer, or about an 8:00/mile. Front of the pack non-elite runners tend to cross the line under 20 minutes, while professional runners are in the 15-minute range for women and the 13- to 14-minute range for men.

Ready to Start Training?

Regardless of your level of experience, all runners training for a 5k need to remember that even though it's a relatively short race, it's still highly aerobic. Aerobic means that you are using oxygen to unlock the fuel in your cells to move your muscles. The way you build a big aerobic engine is lots of slow running or even walking.

Now when I say, "lots of slow running," that's relative to your experience and fitness level. If you've never run before, popping out the door for a three-mile jog will land you right back on the couch where you started.

But for an everyday runner, three miles a day might be your sweet spot or might not be much at all. Again, the details depend on where you are starting from, but the advice is the same: Spend most of your training staying in the aerobic zone where you can talk easily but are still moving your body.

Run/Walk

If you are a brand-new runner and are not coming from another sport, just covering the distance of three miles could be a lot for you, and that's okay. We all have to start somewhere.

For these runners, I recommend a run/walk program. So you might walk for five minutes as your warm-up, then run for two minutes, and then walk for two minutes. You could repeat this sequence for 20 or 30 minutes and then finish with a walk to cool down. Then on day two, I recommend resting or just walking. On day three, try adding a minute to your run segments. Then the next day, rest or just walk.

After a couple of weeks, you could be fit enough to lengthen your runs into miles instead of minutes, always making sure that you are recovering well between workouts to build up your muscles and prevent injury. If you are sore or extra tired, give yourself an extra rest day or go back to a run/walk sequence.

Eventually, you'll be able to run three miles in training, and, if you like, you can go ahead and sign up for your first 5k to see what the race experience is like.

Add Some Speed

Once you are comfortable with the distance, you'll want to work on your speed. And more specifically than just raw speed, you want to work on your stamina, which is the combination of speed and endurance.

You could go out to your local track and bust out some short repeats as fast as you can, and a lot of people do this. High effort, intense intervals will help you sharpen your raw speed, but they don't give you what you really need, which is the ability to sustain your speed over 3.1 miles. So for that, we need to get specific.

Six Weeks of 5k-Specific Workouts

A perfect workout to prepare specifically for the 5k is 12 repeats of 400 meters, or a quarter mile at your goal 5k pace with short but relatively quick jogging the rest of the 100 meters. No stopping or walking if you can help it.

If you don't know what your goal pace is, try to pick a pace that would be a medium-hard effort for a quarter mile but nowhere near all out, perhaps a 6 or a 7 on a scale of 1 to 10. You want to find a speed you can sustain the whole workout without burning out and still be able to keep those jog breaks honest.

By the time you are done, you have just run a 5k at your goal pace (well, technically 4800 meters), and you did it with very little recovery.

By not fully recovering and jogging quickly between repeats, you still improve your ability to run at race pace, but you ensure that you have the aerobic strength and support to maintain goal pace on race day.

The following week do the same thing, but do it with 600s (so that would be 8x600 meters at goal pace with 200 meters of jogging in between).

The next week is 6x800, so now you are up to a half mile at a time at goal pace.

By week four, it might be time to test yourself a little and see if you have improved over the last month, so go ahead and do the 400 workout again, but this time, spice it up a little and hit the gas on the last interval or the second to last interval. This teaches you that you can work even harder at the end of a workout when you are tired, which is definitely something that you will need on race day.

Then, on week five, try the 800 workout again, and see if you can drop the hammer on the last interval there.

By week six, you should be just about ready to race that weekend. You want to keep your legs sharp by including some speed about five days ahead of the race but not so much that you are tired on race day.

A good race week workout could be a mile at faster than 5k goal pace, rest for three to five minutes, and then a couple of 400s faster than race pace. While going faster than goal seems counterintuitive, your fitness is already built by now, and you are just reinforcing the connection between your brain and your legs for this one. The other reason faster than goal is good here is because it makes your real goal pace feel way more comfortable!

If you are a very advanced runner, you can probably handle more reps than what I've outlined, but the structure is exactly the same—chop up the 5k into little pieces separated by short, quick jogs.

Of course, all of the workouts I've just described include a good warm-up and cool-down of nice and easy running of a length that's appropriate for your experience.

And also, no runner's training would be complete without proper rest and recovery as well as just enough strength training to keep the body strong and injury free.

Race Day

The 5k has the reputation of being a lung-searing, quad-burning race where you start fast, stay fast in the middle, and speed up towards the end. And that's pretty much exactly the strategy for racing it.

As with all endurance races, running negative splits or finishing faster than you started is the recommended strategy for most 5k courses (see the "Race Strategy" section). If you are running it hard, it will hurt, but thankfully it's over quickly, and you can be recovered enough to race it again the following weekend.

The Half Marathon

A half marathon is 13.1 miles, or 21 kilometers, and let's face it, it lives in the shadow of its big brother the full marathon. I mean, it doesn't even get its own name! It's just half of something else. Which is truly sad, because it's a great race all on its own.

What's nice about it is that you still have to train for it unless you are just genetically gifted at getting up off the couch and running for 13 miles. But it doesn't completely take over your life like marathon training does. You don't have to sacrifice every Saturday morning for three or four months to be good at the half, and you don't have to run nearly as many miles per day or per week.

If you are a new runner, the idea of running a half is an admirable and worthy goal that's exciting and motivating. After all, not many people choose to run for two hours or more just for fun.

And if you've been slogging away at multiple marathons a year for several years, switching to halves can refresh your legs and your outlook and make marathon pace feel a lot easier.

The buildup for a half will vary depending on your fitness level and lifestyle, but a fit endurance runner can get ready for a half in 6 to 12 weeks as opposed to the 12 to 20 weeks needed for a full marathon.

The Half Is Highly Aerobic

The half is a highly aerobic event, so keeping the majority of your training miles in the easy zone is your best bet. Not only does this build the exact energy system that you will rely most upon during the race, but keeping it slow helps prevent injuries. I like to say that the easy miles are the cake and speed work is the icing. Cake is still pretty good without the icing, but it doesn't really work the other way around.

Build Slowly

If you are just starting out, you'll want to build your weekly miles and your long run miles gradually. The best way to do that is to build for three weeks, then cut back the fourth week, then build again, repeating the third week mileage. This keeps you from adding too much too soon and allows you to absorb all the good training.

For example, if your long run is five miles in week one, you can build to six on week two, seven on week three, go back to five for week four, then go back to seven for week six, building for another three weeks before dropping back again. Ideally, if you're a newer runner, your long run should build to 11 to 13 miles.

If you're a more experienced runner, you will want to build in the same pattern but will be starting from a higher base, so adding two or even three miles to your long run is generally safe and recommended since, percentage-wise, it's not that big of a jump. Veteran runners should aim for a long run of 14 to 16 miles when training for the half.

Add Smart Speed

If you are just looking to finish the distance for the first time or for the first time in a long time, adding speed elements to your long run isn't really necessary. But if you are ready to try to crack that PR, adding a few miles at race pace to the end of your long run is a great idea. For my athletes, I typically add some kind of speed element to the long run every other week.

For your mid-week workouts, and I define a workout as any run that's meant to be faster than easy pace, you can add a shorter interval speed session in the early part of the week and a tempo-type run a couple days later.

But a word of caution with that. Take a look at your weekly runs and be sure that only 20 percent of the time you are running fast. You absolutely can train for a half only running three days a week, but if you do that, it's not a great idea for those to be two speed sessions and a long run. If you do that, you are limiting your ability to develop your aerobic system, which is the majority of what you need for the race.

The best kinds of workouts to get faster for the half marathon borrow from both 5k training and from marathon training. You'll sharpen up your high-end speed with faster (but shorter) 5k workouts, and you'll improve your stamina (speed plus endurance) with marathon-type tempo and threshold workouts.

The only difference is that your paces for the half marathon are going to be faster than for the marathon, so your training paces should be as well. That means you'll be practicing half-marathon paces in half-marathon training and marathon paces in marathon training, but the structure of the workouts are similar.

Should You Cross Train During Half Marathon Training?

Cross training, or engaging in another aerobic activity on a non-running day, can be helpful for those runners who are looking to add more aerobic fitness without the pounding of more miles on the run. While this can work well, if your main priority is running, then that should be your main activity.

What if you run hard or long just three days a week but spend another two or three days on the bike or in the pool? Aren't you working your aerobic system by doing that?

The answer is yes, you are, and there are plenty of programs out there that are designed just like this. They tell you to run hard a couple times a week and then do other things to boost your aerobic system the rest of the time. That might work fine if you are training for a triathlon, but I'll tell you that most triathlon athletes don't train that way either.

The problem with this approach is that the thinking is backwards. The theory is that by running less, you are putting less stress on your bones and joints and you recover while swimming or biking. I agree that you can recover with cross training, but if all you do is run hard less often, you are increasing your chance of injury and slowing your body's time to adapt, because every time you run, you are running hard with lots of stress on non-adapted legs.

Sneak Up on Your Fitness

When you run slow and easy more often, you are sneaking up on your fitness. Your body doesn't even really realize that it's working that hard, because it's not working that hard! But it still makes the little adjustments necessary to make you a more efficient runner. You are not shocking your system by banging out blistering 400-meter repeats once a week.

When you instead run a lot of slow miles most of the time and then turn up the pace for the 400s, your body doesn't freak out and sound the alarm, because it recognizes running, even faster running, as just a normal thing that it's used to.

So if you can only run three days a week, make one of those days nice and slow, and keep the speed work to a sprinkle.

Fueling for the Half

Fueling is another way the half is so much more manageable than the full. Mid-race nutrition is far less critical, but you still need to have a plan.

If you can run a half in less than 90 minutes, you technically don't need to take in any calories during the race. That's because if you ate the night before and had a decent breakfast the morning of, your liver and muscles will have enough glycogen on board to last you the whole time.

But just because you don't have to take in fuel doesn't mean that you shouldn't. Your brain will start to reign in the speed in your legs well before the tank hits zero. In fact, some studies show that performance declines when the muscles still have half of their glycogen capacity stored. You can work in training on improving this, but it's a lot simpler to take in a few calories of your favorite fuel on the race course. I like to do that early on in the race (about 40 minutes in) to keep my brain happy.

But if you are like most runners, the half will take longer than 90 minutes, and you should plan to take in fuel once or twice during the race. A great timing plan is every 35 to 45 minutes, but be sure to practice your plan on your long runs to be sure that it works for you, because every tummy is different.

Hydrating for the Half

Even if you are running in cool weather, hydration is important for the half marathon. In any run longer than 60 minutes, dehydration can affect how you feel and how you perform. See chapter four for more details on crafting a hydration plan for you.

The half marathon is an awesome distance that is challenging yet still allows you to have a normal life. Well, that is until you get so good at them that you decide to step it up to the full...

Training for a Marathon

If you've run a half or two, you might have started to think about training for a marathon. In this section, I explore the details of marathon training and specifically how long it takes to be ready to handle the demands of 26.2 miles.

How Long Do You Need to Train?

If you jump on Google and search for marathon training plans, you'll see that most plans are between 12 and 20 weeks. And that might be right for some people, but that's definitely not a good idea for everyone. So how do you know if that's right for you?

As a coach, the first thing I look at is experience. There's a big difference between someone who's just starting out and someone who has regularly run most days of the week for years. Running 26.2 miles puts an immense amount of strain on your muscles, bones, and tendons, and if you haven't toughened them up from years of running, you should definitely be cautious before signing up for your first marathon.

Beginners

So let's say that you are an absolute beginner. You've gotten up off the couch and bought your first pair of running shoes and gone out for a couple of runs. How long will it take you to become a marathoner?

Well, if you are at that stage, a marathon is not what you should be focusing on at first. If a race atmosphere inspires you, then aiming for running your first 5k or 3.1 miles is a perfect way to test out the running waters. If the thought of racing a 5k doesn't inspire you, though, you don't have to take all the race distance steps in order, but you still have to take your time to build up to long distance running.

It would be really logical to tell you to start with a 5k, then move up to 10k, then train for a half, and then get ready for the marathon. Honestly, that's probably the best way to do it, and it's what the majority of elite runners do. But I know that runners can be an impatient bunch, wanting results immediately. The marathon has an allure to it that the 5k just doesn't have, so I get that people want to go for the glory right away.

But I would certainly recommend racing a half before racing a full. A huge part of racing well is experience at racing, not just running, so knowing a bit about what to expect will make a huge difference in how your first marathon goes.

But let's say you want to ignore that advice and go straight from the couch to the marathon with zero races in between. If you are going to do that, I would recommend that you at least build your weekly long run up to 8 to 10 miles before starting a true marathon training buildup. Once you are there, I'd recommend at least 20 weeks of training before the big day.

Casual and Intermediate Runners

Now what if you aren't completely starting from scratch? Maybe you've run casually for a while now. Perhaps you've already run a few races or even a marathon a few years ago. You're not starting from zero, but you are not in marathon shape either. In that case, you might not need a full 20 weeks, but 18 weeks is a really good idea.

Next, let's talk about the intermediate runners. These are the runners that run consistently three to five times a week and get up to 25 to 35 miles per week and typically have long runs of 10 miles or longer each week.

These runners already have a solid base of running and are probably focused on running a marathon faster than before, not just completing it. So it's not just about building up more mileage to be able to handle the distance, it's about maximizing performance. A good marathon training plan for these runners will be between 14 to 18 weeks and will include long runs that are not just long but also have an element of speed in them such as a fast finish long run.

I will say that it is very challenging to be adequately prepared for a marathon by running three days or fewer a week with fewer than 30 miles per week. It's not that it can't be done (people do it all the time), but your body will suffer a lot more on race day and during training.

It's also really shocking to your system to have a 20 mile long run on your schedule when you are only running 5 miles two other days of the week. Keeping your mileage buildup smooth not only from week to week but throughout your weeks is key to sneaking up on your fitness rather than forcing it.

Advanced Runners

Now let's talk about advanced runners. A lot of advanced runners I know hate to be called advanced, because while they run all the time and are in great shape, they are nowhere near elite level. But we're not talking about the pros here. An advanced runner is someone who runs more than four days and 40 miles a week and can easily run 12 to 15 miles for a long run.

These runners will not need as much time to specifically train for a marathon. They already have a good running foundation, which is at the heart of the first phase of a longer marathon build. An advanced marathoner can get away with 12 weeks of specific marathon training. The goal is to run the marathon as fast as they can.

Just like the intermediate runner, the advanced runner will focus on increasing the length of the long run for the first part of the build and then will spend a good chunk of time working on their speed endurance, also known as stamina. The long runs can be a bit longer than an intermediate's, and many of their long runs will have speed elements to them to be as close as possible to what they will experience on race day.

Marathon Junkies

And finally, we have those runners who race all the time. These are the marathon maniacs or ultramarathoners who race several very long races a year and sometimes a couple in the same month. How long should they take between each race?

Well, this is kind of a tricky one. There is a lot of good science that says that muscle recovery isn't fully complete until three weeks after the marathon and presumably longer for anything longer than that. So while they might be back to baseline three weeks after a race, that doesn't leave any time left to build and improve. That takes many weeks or even months, which is why most elites only race two marathons a year. There are, of course, elites that race marathons more often than that, but that's more of the exception rather than the rule.

So if you simply love racing marathons and ultras, and major improvement is not your goal, you can do several in a single year as long as you take the time to recover to avoid an injury that sends you back to the couch. Because then you'll have to start all over again.

Marathon-Specific Runs and Workouts

Following are specific runs and workouts design to help you train for a marathon.

Once you get past the half marathon distance, it's no longer beneficial to run the distance of your race in training. In fact, many new runners can be successful at the marathon with a long run topping out at only 16 miles (25.75km).

That can be hard to grasp for a new runner. After all, how do you know that you actually CAN run the marathon if you have never run it in training?

The reason you do not want to run very long runs in training is that each time you run longer than about three hours, you start to get diminishing returns. The aerobic benefit, which is the primary reason for running long, starts to decline, while your injury risk begins to rise. Recent science has shown that a run longer than three hours is no better for your development than one of two and a half hours!

Not to mention, you'll need a lot more time to recover from a 22-miler than you would need for a shorter long run, which potentially means sacrificing other helpful runs while you rest.

So instead of planning long runs beyond three hours, it is far better to do a shorter steady run the day before the long run. That way, you will be beginning your long run with tired legs and not starting from zero.

For example, you might run an 8-mile steady run, which is medium-effort paced (neither easy nor hard) on a Friday and then a long run of 16 miles on Saturday, totaling 24 miles in two days. You will not feel as fresh for the long run, and it's as if you are really starting at mile eight when you factor in the day before.

This concept of "pre-fatiguing" your legs allows for a better and shorter long run at faster paces, better physiological training, and quicker recovery. You will build your tolerance for running on tired legs through accumulated fatigue, which is exactly what you will need on race day.

Fast Finish Long Runs

Being able to run fast on tired legs is key to racing your best race in any distance, and it's especially important in the marathon. Practicing finishing fast at the end of a long run will train your body and your brain that you can do it on race day with confidence.

How to Run a Fast Finish Long Run

It's best to schedule a fast finish long run every other long run once you've established a good base mileage for your long run. That can be 14 to 16 miles, but of course, this number is different for every runner.

To use an 18-mile run as an example, you'll start off at an easy pace, where you could talk comfortably the entire time with a running buddy. Keep it easy for 13 miles, and resist the temptation to go too fast.

Then, for the next three miles, you'll want to speed up to a "comfortably hard pace," which is usually around 10 to 15 seconds faster than your estimated marathon pace. For example, a four-hour marathoner would aim for a pace of around 8:55-9:00 minutes per mile for the three fast miles. If the first two speedy miles feel pretty good, you can gradually push the pace a bit until you are running as hard as you can sustain for the rest of that mile.

When your watch hits 16 miles, slow down to your easy run pace for the final 2 miles as a "sort-of" cool-down. Don't stop unless you absolutely need to.

Fast finish long runs, in combination with steady runs before the long run, help simulate late-race fatigue while being more specific to energy demands of the race compared with traditional long and slow runs.

Fast finish long runs are tough! So don't do them every single week. Always alternate an easier, slower long run every other week to minimize your injury risk while keeping up your aerobic fitness.

Long Runs With Surges

Adding little bursts of speed to a long run can help better prepare you for your race without making the run too much more difficult. The majority of the long run is still done at your easy aerobic pace, but adding a few surges of speed can spice things up.

Much like how strides (see the Strides section in chapter five) help you run faster with small pieces of speed, surges in a long run can add faster running without disrupting a good 80/20 running ratio of easy to fast. Like the fast finish long run, the surge run teaches you to run fast while fatigued, which develops race-specific strength and skills.

Speed training in general helps improve running mechanics, increases efficiency, and prepares your body for race pace or faster efforts. By sneaking a little speed into some of your other runs, you are getting the benefits of speedwork without the risks.

Surges also help you mentally prepare for the race. As the marathon goes on, you will feel increasingly more tired, and the effort will go up, even if you are maintaining the same pace. But when you practice running faster in training while you are tired, you are gaining experience with the skill of running hard when you'd rather slow down.

When you try this run, you will likely discover two things. Number one is that the first surge is always the hardest, and number two is that when you slow back down to your normal long run pace, you will find your "easy" pace is now faster than before the surge.

The reason that the first surge feels the hardest is because your body gets "pace-locked," or accustomed to whatever pace you've been running. When you change paces, your body needs time to adjust and might protest! This can happen in either direction, so slowing down at the right time can be just or nearly as difficult.

How to Run a Long Run With Surges

Long run surges should begin about halfway through the long run and end about 75 to 80 percent of the way through the run.

For example, if you have a 10-mile-long run that usually takes you 1 hour and 40 minutes to complete, and you're scheduled for 5x1 minute surges with 5 minutes of jogging in between, you should begin the surges at mile five, which will result in the last surge occurring at around mile eight. The length of the surge itself, the rest in between the interval, and the starting point of the surge during the run are all variables that you can adjust to make the workout harder or easier.

The pace should be much faster than marathon pace, or around 5-10k pace. If you don't know your race paces, aim for a "challenging but doable" effort.

Tempo and Threshold Runs

A tempo run, or a threshold run, is a classic workout for long distance runners with a lot of benefits and a lot of confusing terms. Let's clear that up!

Running is a lot like baking a cake. With the right ingredients, the right tools, the right recipe, and some experience in the kitchen, you can craft a restaurant-worthy gourmet dessert. On the other hand, if you simply throw together a bunch of random things in a blender and pop it in the oven, you might get something edible, but it's highly unlikely that it's going to be amazing. Following a recipe with quality ingredients will have a far higher chance of success.

The same is true for endurance running. There are plenty of ingredients, recipes, and tools for creating a great race experience, and no one method is superior for every runner. But there are some tried and true ingredients that come up again and again because they are so useful and effective. Just like staples in your pantry, there are staple workouts that you'll want to stock up on.

One of the most fundamental groups of staple workouts are tempo runs. Tempo runs have quite a few flavors, so I'll go over the different variations and names. I'll get into when to use it, how often, and when to add a little spice.

What Are Tempo Runs?

The simplest way to describe a tempo is "a sustained effort for a specific period of time." It is harder than easy, but not too hard. Now that's not very scientific, which is going to bother those runners out there that love all the data!

But actually, this definition really hits the spirit or the goal of the tempo perfectly well: You are running hard, but not too hard, for a specific amount of time, with the goal of increasing the amount of time you can run at that pace.

Let's look a little deeper at what's going on, because that will tell us how best to use this ingredient in a runner's recipe and in what amount.

The Three Thresholds of Tempo Runs

There are three main phases of intensity when it comes to running that all play a key role in determining how you should run your tempo: aerobic threshold, lactate threshold, and anaerobic threshold. To make things more confusing, these are often used interchangeably, so we'll go through each one so you can be the smartest one at your next group run.

1. Aerobic Threshold

When you run at an easy pace, the effort is called aerobic, meaning with oxygen. Your aerobic system is the main energy system used in long distance running, so you'll want to develop it well to get better at endurance running.

I like to call easy running the cake and everything else the frosting and the decoration. The cake is clearly the most important part and can stand alone as a pretty great dessert. But some frosting (or faster endurance running) and a few fancy sprinkles take the cake to the next level.

Once you start to run harder than an easy pace, there will be a certain point when the effort starts to get more challenging. Your body will start to shift from happily using oxygen to burn fat, protein, and carbohydrate and will start to build up lactic acid in the bloodstream. Your aerobic threshold is the highest level of exercise intensity at which you can run without accumulating significant lactic acid in the blood. For most runners, this is roughly your current marathon race pace.

So how can you make sure that you are running the right pace to increase your aerobic threshold? A good rule of thumb for those without a definable marathon race pace is the target heart rate zone of 60 to 80 percent of maximum heart rate.

Another way to sneak in some aerobic threshold work is to drizzle in a few miles of marathon pace into some of your long runs. I also love adding a steady run the day before your long run, which is about marathon pace, or up to 30 seconds per mile slower.

This not only sneaks in a little more marathon pace practice, but it also pre-fatigues your legs for the next run. That makes your long run feel a little bit harder, but it also allows you to shorten the long run to under three hours, providing the maximum benefit with the least amount of risk and recovery time.

2. Lactate Threshold

But once the leg-burning lactic acid starts to build up, you've reached the lactate threshold. In this zone, your body can still clear away the lactic acid up to a point or even use the lactate as fuel. But, if you keep running at that same challenging pace or perhaps even speed up, you'll cross over into the anaerobic threshold.

Lactic acid and lactate are sometimes used interchangeably even though they are technically different. Lactic acid is the joining of lactate with a hydrogen ion. It's the hydrogen ion in the lactic acid that contributes to the burning sensation in the muscles during exercise, not the lactate. The slowdown in your pace is your body's way of protecting itself from a dangerous rise in acidity in the muscles, or acidosis.

Lactate can get recycled back into our system to provide energy for our muscles, so it is not a bad thing.

3. Anaerobic Threshold

This describes the point at which lactic acid builds faster than the body is able to remove it, and it won't take long before you are forced to slow down.

For most runners, this pace will be about what you can run for 60 minutes in a race environment. So if you are a 60 minute 10k runner, your 10k pace will be your anaerobic threshold pace.

Now that doesn't mean that you want to actually go out and run for 60 minutes as hard as you can and call it a tempo! You'll want to break that down into manageable pieces so you are not "racing your training."

Focus on Current Fitness Instead of Goal Pace

One important thing to remember is that when we talk about race paces or even goal paces, what we really want to do is train at our current pace, not what we hope to achieve. You might have an amazing race goal, and I'm all for big goals, but your level of fitness in training might not match that just yet. So if you are targeting a goal marathon pace in your workouts and you continually end up crossing that lactate threshold line, you're going to end up undermining your training.

If you are a marathoner, the idea is to raise our happy and efficient aerobic threshold as high as possible. That will ensure you can run the entire marathon distance as fast as possible without being forced to slow down when your anaerobic system runs out of gas.

And while aerobic capacity is king in endurance running, you will also want to push the lactate and anaerobic thresholds back, teaching your body to better clear lactic acid when it builds so you can use it as fuel. That means some of your tempo runs should be fast enough to build up lactic acid and cross that threshold.

Effort Is More Important Than Pace

Overall, when it comes to tempos, or really any kind of running workout, your actual pace in training is far less important than your effort. If it's hot and humid, you are going to build up lactic acid at a far slower running speed than you would in perfect conditions. If you don't slow your pace accordingly, you will end up crossing into the anaerobic zone when you were trying to target your aerobic threshold.

That doesn't always mean you've ruined your cake; you're just not following the recipe. But you also don't always have to be so scientific about it. Paces can be a nice guide, but it always has to be about effort.

Know The Why Behind Your Workout

Understanding why you are running specific types of workouts is incredibly helpful to get the effort level intended to get the results that you are looking for. It's easy to overcomplicate things by adding in new ingredients in an effort to improve. But more often than not, simple, quality ingredients in just the right amount along with a great recipe will make a far better cake. And a better runner.

Tempo Intervals

Whether you are a beginner or an experienced marathoner, jumping straight into big tempo runs early in your training cycle is probably going to be too much too soon. A better way of getting to the speeds that you are hoping for is to break up the tempos into smaller efforts.

How to Run Tempo Intervals

After a mile or two of easy jogging as a warm-up, start off with a mile or five minutes at your aerobic or lactate threshold pace. This will feel "comfortably hard," yet you are in control and are holding some effort back.

Once you reach the end of your interval, jog easy for a minute or two. Repeat as many times as your fitness level suggests. Beginners might start with two or three intervals.

The idea is to get a "speed spike" and cross the threshold line, then bring it back down. This allows you to spend more time at higher speeds with great form while not pushing your limits too far and risking injury.

Finish with a mile or two of easy jogging as a cool-down. An example of a tempo interval workout for a runner with a four-hour marathon fitness level would be a 1-mile jogging warm-up, 3x2 miles at 8:50-9:00 pace with four minutes of rest, and a 1-mile jogging cool-down.

The Basic Tempo

Once you get comfortable getting a little uncomfortable with tempo intervals, you can try running at your tempo speed in one big chunk. This will teach your body to adapt to longer periods of faster running. For most people, a tempo run is faster than their marathon pace, and it will help you feel like marathon pace is much easier!

How to Run the Basic Tempo

After a mile or two of easy jogging as a warm-up, speed up to your aerobic or lactate threshold pace and hang on to it for three to eight miles, depending on your fitness level.

Finish with a mile or two of easy jogging as a cool-down.

An example of a basic tempo run for a runner with a four-hour marathon fitness level would be a 2-mile jogging warm-up, 4 miles at 8:50-9:00 pace with four minutes of rest, and a 2-mile jogging cool-down.

Cutdown Runs

A cutdown run, also called a progression run, is where you progressively get faster, or cut down your pace with each mile.

Cutdowns are an especially important training tool for the marathon and the half marathon because they teach the brain and the legs that you can increase your effort and your speed despite getting more and more tired.

The key to a successful cutdown is not simply to aim to get faster every mile. To do it right, you have to purposely slow down, or sandbag, the first few miles. In fact, learning to sandbag is an incredibly important skill for all your workouts and races. That's because your effort always increases with the time you spend running hard. It's far better and easier to control your effort at the beginning and increase as you go rather than starting off too fast and being forced to slow with exhaustion.

After all, speed is only useful when you can control it!

When you practice starting easy then speeding up, you are simulating what you will feel on race day. Set yourself up for race day success with cutdown tempos in training!

How to Run a Cutdown

After a mile or two of easy jogging to warm up, begin your first cutdown mile. This first mile should be faster than your easy pace, but not by much. Typically, it would be 20 to 30 seconds slower than your marathon pace. If you don't know your marathon pace, aim to start about 10 to 20 seconds per mile faster than what you would run for a nice and slow warm-up.

Each consecutive mile, cut down your pace (i.e., speed up) by ten seconds per mile. As always, the length of your workout will depend on your fitness level and mileage. Your final mile should feel very challenging (usually a bit faster than half marathon pace), but not so challenging that you have to slow down or stop.

Finish with a mile or two of easy jogging as a cool-down.

This is not an easy run, but with practice you will get better at it. Once race day comes along, you will instinctively know how to increase your effort and push harder to maintain your pace.

An example cutdown workout for someone who is fit enough to run four hours for the marathon would look something like this: one-mile warm-up, six-mile cutdown run (9:45, 9:35, 9:25, 9:15, 9:05, 8:55), and a one-mile cool-down.

Alternating Tempos

Alternating tempos (AT) are a more advanced marathon and half marathon training run, so it's a good idea to have a few basic tempos and cutdowns behind you before trying the AT.

When we start to run faster, our bodies can only "clear," or reconvert, a certain amount of lactic acid into energy before fatigue strikes. If we want to race faster, we must teach our body to process it more efficiently.

The basic tempo run and tempo intervals help your body improve this process by gradually increasing the level of lactate in your system. You slowly adapt to the increased lactic acid levels and eventually can run faster longer.

But if you can flood the body with lactic acid by running at a fast pace and then drop back to half-marathon or marathon pace to "recover," your body will learn to deal with the rising levels of lactic acid more efficiently while running fast. This means that you can more effectively use lactate as a fuel source and run faster and farther without getting as tired.

How to Run an Alternating Tempo

It's important to remember that in all your workouts, faster is not better. This is especially true with the AT. You need to be running two distinct speeds, fast and faster, to nail the purpose.

After a mile or two of easy jogging to warm up, begin your first mile. This should be your faster pace to begin to flood your system with lactic acid. It will be between half marathon and 10k race pace for most runners. If you don't know your race paces, it will be very challenging, yet not even close to all-out. Once you finish that faster mile, drop down to a still fast but more comfortable pace. For most runners, that's just a little faster than marathon pace.

Repeat the alternating faster/fast miles for a total of four to six miles, depending on your fitness level. Finish with a mile or two of easy jogging as a cool-down.

An example for a fit 3:30 marathon runner, the alternating tempo would look like this: one- to three-mile jogging warm-up, six miles at 7:50, 7:25, 7:50, 7:25, 7:50, 7:25 with no rest, and a one- to two-mile jogging cool-down.

5k and Faster Speedwork for Marathoners

Keira D'Amato, the American record holder in the marathon, doesn't just train "like a marathoner." As she told me when I interviewed her for the Run to the Top Podcast in December 2020, she also trains like a 5k runner. She says this faster training once a week is what has propelled her into the record books at all distances.

Along with marathon-specific work like long runs and tempos, adding in 5k workouts once a week or every 10 days can raise your level of fitness. This not only makes

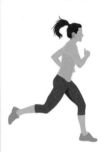

SIX WEEKS OF 5K SPECIFIC WORKOUTS

The goal of 5k workouts is to chop up the 3.1 mile race into pieces with jogging breaks. You are practicing race goal pace and distance in managable bites. If you don't know your 5k pace, aim for a medium hard effort.

WEEK ONE: 12 reps of 400 meters with 100 meter jog rests

WEEK TWO: 8 reps of 600m with 200m jog rests

WEEK THREE: 6 reps of 800m with 200m jog rests

WEEK FOUR: 12 reps of 400m with 100m jog rests, hammer #11 almost as fast as you can

WEEK FIVE: 6 reps of 800m with 200m jog rests, hammer #5 almost as fast as you can

WEEK SIX (RACE WEEK): 1 mile, 200m jog rest, 2 reps of 400m. Paces can be slightly faster to "wake up" the legs!

the **planted** *runner*

marathon-pace running feel easier but will help you to become more efficient at all speeds.

Be sure that you schedule enough recovery time between your track sessions, tempos, and long runs. Many fit runners under 40 who are running five days a week or more can handle one of each of these hard sessions a week. Beginners and older runners may find that spreading out these workouts over 10 days better allows for the proper amount of recovery time.

Tapering Down

As you get closer to race day, you'll want to begin tapering off your training so that you start on the line fresh and fast. Your longest long run should be scheduled three weeks away from race day, and the next two long runs should get progressively shorter.

The final three weeks of training before the marathon will do little to improve your fitness level since it's already built. But you certainly can harm your fitness in those weeks, so when in doubt, less is more!

Taper Workouts

During taper, your overall weekly mileage should decrease 10 to 20 percent per week. But don't stop running completely or change your frequency of running. Your body hates sudden and drastic changes, so ease into it.

Your workouts during taper should all be about practicing your marathon goal pace in various types of tempos. This is to burn marathon pace into your muscle memory so that it becomes second nature and your confidence builds.

This period of time will also help tell you if your marathon pace goal is realistic. If your marathon paced tempos during tempo feel far too hard, you are probably being too aggressive with your goal. Marathon pace should not feel easy unless this is your very first one, but it should not be super challenging for just a few miles. You can learn more about ways to tell if you are ready for the marathon later in this chapter.

An example of a taper workout would be a 6-mile marathon pace tempo in the third week before the race, a 2x3 mile tempo in the second week, and a 3-mile marathon pace tempo in race week. These all, of course, will also include a mile or two of easy jogging for both the warm-up and the cool-down.

The day before the race, a 15-minute slow jog is perfect to get the blood moving without expending too much energy.

When To Back Off Strength Training

Again, you should not be trying to change things up too much from normal during taper, just backing off the length and intensity. So if you normally strength train twice a week, you should still do that for a while, but your routine should be shorter, with fewer reps and lighter weights (if any). You should never lift to fatigue during taper.

Stop strength training completely 10 days before your race. Fitness gains from strength work do not realize for about 10 days, and you don't want to risk fatigue from lifting. Remember, you will not gain any fitness taper week. You are simply going through the motions so that your body is tricked into thinking everything's normal.

You Might Not Feel Better During Taper

Some of us just don't feel good during taper. Some people even start to get sick because the immune system lets its guard down after months of hard training. Not feeling great happens to a lot of us because it takes 10 to 12 days to fully recover from hard workouts[34], which means you are not going to suddenly feel fresh and peppy.

Should I Schedule a Massage?

Be careful with this one. If you normally get weekly massages (lucky you!), then staying with your routine is probably the best plan, as long as you let your therapist know to take it easy on you this week. But if you do not have a regular massage routine, this is not the time to start. Massages are wonderful, but they can also leave you sore, which is the opposite of what you want.

How Can I Tell If I'm Ready for My Marathon Goal Pace?

Most first-time marathoners are just happy to be able to finish a marathon, but once you have that first one behind you, almost everyone wants to know if it can be done faster.

The quick answer to that question is, no one knows! You can be the most highly trained elite marathoner in the world, and if you have a terrible day, you might not make it to the finish line. That's just the harsh reality of the race. You train for months on end, and it ends up being a crap shoot on just one single day. But let's assume that weather is not a major factor. How do you know that you've done enough to prepare yourself for what you think you can accomplish?

For anything but your very first marathon, where you are simply trying to finish, goal marathon pace should feel a step harder than easy. The more experienced you are at the marathon, the more you can push the effort level. If you've had a good buildup, goal pace should be something that felt pretty hard the first few weeks, more manageable in the middle, and good (but still a little scary) toward the end.

There are seven major signs that you are ready to race the marathon.

1 Consistency Matters More Than Perfection

The first thing to do is look back at your training log. How consistent were you with your mileage and fitting in your runs? Consistency is, hands down, the single most important aspect of good training. Running stable mileage without big gaps in training or big swings in mileage is key to being well prepared. Your runs don't all have to be Facebook-worthy; just showing up day after day is what matters most.

2 Solid Long Runs

The second thing I look at as a coach is your long runs. Did you get all or most of them in? Did the majority of them go well, or were you strapped to the struggle bus the whole time? Simply running long at a slow pace does tremendous things for your aerobic system, but adding the extra challenge of some speed to a long run can really test your legs for the big day. Fast finish long runs are great at signaling how you might hold up in the marathon, especially if you paired the run with a moderately paced steady run the day before and still survived. Teaching yourself to keep running hard when tired is exactly the skill you will need on race day, so if you have a time goal in mind, you definitely need to practice this!

3 Prioritizing Recovery

The next thing I want to know is how well you are recovering from those hard days and those long, hard runs. Are you able to run easy the next day with minimal to no soreness in the last few weeks before the race? Or do you have to take extra recovery time to get to feeling like yourself again? At the beginning of your training cycle, it's very normal to have leg soreness after hard workouts, but the goal is to build strong legs that can handle what the marathon has to throw at you. A well-designed training plan will build tough, durable legs that can go the distance without being completely trashed the next day.

4 Goal Pace Starts to Feel Pretty Good

Number four might seem overly obvious: How does goal pace feel? At the beginning of the cycle, a few miles at race pace typically feels on the harder side, but as you get closer to the race, goal pace should start feeling pretty good. It's certainly still significantly harder than easy pace, but it should not be a struggle to maintain it for several miles. After all, you are going to be running at that pace for hours! If you are sucking wind after 30 minutes and it's three weeks before your race, it's highly likely that your goal is far too aggressive.

5 Fueling and Hydration

The next factor in the equation is fueling and hydration. Have you found what works for you and practiced it until it's second nature? Nearly all of your long runs and many of your later-stage fast workouts should be done fully fueled to practice your race day nutrition, including what you will eat the night before the race. Nutrition is what makes marathons more than twice as hard as halves. If you skimp on this section and don't have a well-practiced plan for the race, you could be in big trouble.

6 Healthy at the Starting Line

As a coach, I also want to determine how healthy you are. Are there any lingering injuries that you've been pushing through that haven't properly healed? Have you been truly honest with me and with yourself about how severe an injury is? Athletes are strong, stubborn people, and we don't want anything, especially a little injury, to get in the way of running. But if you neglected to take care of a tweak, a niggle, or an ouch with proper recovery, then pushing harder than you've ever gone before on race day is a huge risk that might not be worth the potential reward.

7 Mental Strength

The last factor is arguably the most important of all: How well have you trained your brain? If you want to reach your potential, you have to dig down into a part of yourself that is a little dark and a little uncomfortable. Running hard for hours on end is no cake walk, and if you don't want it bad enough, all the safety features that your brain has at its disposal to keep you from dying will come out in full force. You run hard in workouts not only to build your physical strength but also to see if you've got what it takes to push past the point where reasonable people slow down or stop.

Now to do that in real life takes discipline that is 100 percent mental. Your brain has to override the feelings of excitement and adrenaline at the beginning of the race to keep your pace under control. You have to learn to stay calm when you see a split that you don't like on your watch and remember that the first 20 miles is just a warm-up for the real race. You have to let go of fears of failure and follow your plan. You have to prepare yourself ahead of time that the last 5-10k of the race will be very, very, very hard if you are doing it right, but you will keep running anyway.

So if nearly everything I've said sounds like you, then you probably have a realistic goal in mind. If none or only a few of the points I've mentioned are true, then it's time to take a step back and rethink your goals. After all, would you rather cross the finish line with a smile on your face knowing you ran the best race you could or skeleton walk the last 10 miles in pure agony because you overshot your goal?

Making a realistic plan for your race is essential to finishing the marathon with a performance you can be proud of.

How to Fuel for the Marathon

Proper fueling for the marathon can be the difference between the race of your life and a disaster. By learning exactly what your body needs to power through the race, you can come up with a fueling plan that you can rely on to run your best race yet!

I'll go into the details of what and how much to eat, but please note that you do not have to count calories or macros to be successful at your marathon fueling! Tracking can be helpful occasionally to get an idea of what you are eating, but I don't recommend it long term.

Race Week (aka Taper Week) Fueling

Taper week can do some crazy things to runners. Some people feel nervous and anxious about the big day. Without as much running scheduled to ease the mind, nerves can get a bit frazzled. We worry about losing fitness and gaining weight, we obsessively stalk the weather forecast, and we stress about making sure every last detail is taken care of.

We get the taper tantrums.

But with some good planning, you can maximize your time and your nutrition so that you are at your best on race day. In general, you want to slightly decrease calories while keeping up the carbs. Because you are running far less in taper week than you did in training, you won't need as many calories.

A mistake many marathoners make is not easing up on how much they eat even though they are burning significantly fewer calories. Definitely eat when you are hungry, but be conscious of eating a little lighter.

Your nutrition goal during taper is to load up your muscle glycogen stores without gaining fat from eating more and running less. You should actually gain weight during taper, but ideally that's from the extra glycogen and water that you are storing, not fat. Having plenty of fuel and hydration stored inside your body before the race is the goal! Don't be alarmed if you gain two to four pounds while carbo-loading.

Carbs Are Your Friends

The goal for carbohydrates should be to maintain a daily intake of three to five grams per pound of body weight. For a 150-pound athlete, this will be approximately 450 to 750 grams (1800 to 3000 calories).

That is a lot of calories and a big range, so be sure to find a number that is relative to your overall caloric needs based on your body size and how much you run.

Protein Is Still Important

While you are loading up on carbs, don't forget about the protein. Protein is needed to repair and reverse muscle damage and fatigue resulting from all your training. Athletes need more protein than sedentary people, so your goal is approximately 0.6 to 0.7 gram per pound of bodyweight. Going back to our example of the 150-pound athlete, this would be 90 to 105 grams of protein per day. This can easily be achieved by having a couple of servings of protein-rich foods.

Many of your carb sources, like grains and beans, provide protein as well. One serving of pasta has about 42 grams of carbohydrate and 7 grams of protein. One slice of whole-grain bread has about 20 grams of carbohydrate and 4 grams of protein.

What About Fat?

In order to decrease calories but keep up carbohydrate intake, you will have to trade some of the calories coming from fat for more carbohydrates. Good fat should still contribute 20 to 25 percent of your total daily calories, but since you will be eating fewer calories, this will mean fewer total grams from fat.

Here are a few examples of some swaps you can make to cut down on fat and increase carbohydrate:

- Pancakes with maple syrup instead of avocado toast
- Pasta with tomato sauce instead of creamy sauce
- Vegetable salad with an extra dinner roll and vinaigrette instead of full-fat dressing
- And my favorite: an extra plain baked potato with salsa or ketchup instead of fatty toppings

Taper Off the Fiber

While fiber is an essential part of any healthy diet, you'll want to taper off high-fiber foods as you get closer to race day.

Foods like white rice and potatoes are perfect in the two days leading up to the race to be sure they are easily digested.

Pre-Hydration

Now let's talk about hydration. We know that dehydration can significantly impair performance, but it is preventable with adequate hydration in the weeks, days, and hours leading up to the race.

To ensure you are properly hydrated, sip on fluids throughout the day. Water is sufficient, but juices and sports drinks can help meet your carbohydrate needs if you are struggling to get all your carbs from food. Adding salt and other electrolytes to your water or adding a little extra salt to your food can also help you retain water, which is normally a bad thing but is great for marathoners.

Hydration needs are drastically individual, so there's no magic number that's right for everyone. (See chapter four for more details.) Drink when you are thirsty, but be sure that you are urinating every two to three hours and that your urine is pale yellow. If it is darker, then hydrate more. If it is clear, you may be hydrating too much. Overdrinking is a real issue for marathon runners, so don't overdo it.

The Day Before the Race

The day before the race, it's smart to avoid alcohol. This might seem obvious, but even a small amount of alcohol can lead to dehydration and poor sleep quality. Not what you need right before the big day!

You'll want to eat your biggest meal at lunch, not at dinner. Yes, it's a common tradition to have a big pasta dinner the night before the race, but eating this meal earlier in the day allows plenty of time for digestion. You don't want to be uncomfortably full on race morning, so try eating a big meal earlier and a normal size meal the night before.

Always choose foods you've had before. Now is not the time to try a new type of pasta or sauce just because you are in a new town and heard about the great reviews. It could come back to haunt you!

My favorite pre-race dinner is a plate of plain potatoes with ketchup. I could rely on that anywhere I traveled, and I knew that it would sit well with my stomach the next day!

Race Day

Alright, race day is here. The first rule of racing is NOTHING NEW ON RACE DAY, so this should be a routine you have practiced many times before.

Breakfast

Be sure to eat breakfast two to three hours before the start. Eating breakfast is important because a small meal rich in carbohydrates will help prevent hunger and maintain a normal blood sugar level. Stick with foods that are familiar and those you have been eating throughout your training. If you enjoy coffee, it can be a performance booster and can help things move along your digestive system, so you can use the bathroom in the comfort of your home or hotel and not during the race!

You'll want to sip on water or a sports drink, but again, not so much that you need to use the bathroom during the race. I prefer to get my fluids in early and not drink anything in the hour before the gun goes off.

During the Race

There are many different products on the market that can fuel the marathon. I have several recipes you can try if you like to make your own fuel which can be found in chapter ten, Planted Runner Recipes:

- DIY UCAN
- Homemade Copy Cat GU Gels
- Real Food Gels

I'll go over the traditional approach with gels and sports drinks, but any product containing quick digesting carbohydrates can help fuel your marathon.

Some runners take a gel 15 minutes before start time, and others prefer to wait a bit to fuel. It's often better to take small doses of fuel more often than bigger doses less often; I recommend that you take something in every 30 to 40 minutes.

Rough guidelines are 30 to 90 grams of carbohydrate per hour from a combo of gels and sports drinks, which is about 150 to 350 calories per hour. Bigger runners need more, and smaller runners need less.

The good thing about using sports drinks is that they also contribute to your hydration, but the bad thing is that they might be hard on sensitive stomachs, so be sure you are taking in water as well.

Most people can only digest 60 grams of carbohydrate per hour, so more isn't better, because it could make you feel sick. That's why a steady intake of calories at frequent intervals throughout the race can help while avoiding blood sugar crashes.

It's important to know that anything you take in during the last 20 to 30 minutes won't reach your system in time to be effective. BUT it might be worthwhile to swish something sweet in your mouth and spit it out, especially if you can't handle any more in your stomach at any point. Just the motion of swishing alerts the brain that carbs are coming, so you do get a bit of a boost. But in general, stick to water near the end of the race.

With a solid fueling and nutrition plan stacked on top of months of good training, there's no limit to what you can accomplish on race day!

The Best Strategy to Race Faster: Negative Split

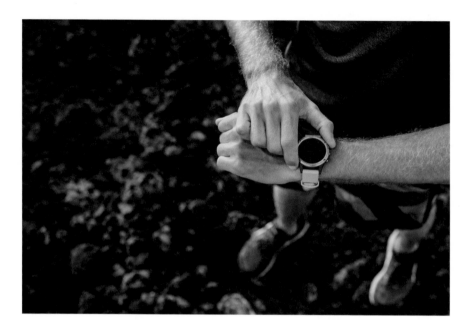

Have you ever watched a little kid run? They blast off as fast as their little legs can go and then flame out to a stop almost as fast as they started.

This instinct to run hard from the start is something that is tough to unlearn. That's why you so often see new runners, and even experienced runners, do the exact same thing in workouts and races. They start off too fast, and at some point dramatically and disappointingly slow down, finishing far slower than their potential.

But there is a proven race strategy that race after race produces far better results. It's a strategy that has led to nearly every world record in distances from 1500 meters to the marathon and beyond. It's called the negative split.

A negative split is simply running the first half of your race slower than your second half. That means you have to run slower when you are feeling good and run faster when you are feeling tired. Sounds impossible, right? Well, it's not easy, for sure, but it's a concept that can work in nearly any race to ensure that you get the very most out of your potential.

Why Going Out Too Fast Will Cost You

It's easy to see why we naturally go out too fast. We feel good and fresh at the start and often underestimate the effort required to sustain our pace through the entire distance. Sure, intellectually we know that the race will get tougher the longer it goes on, but in the quest to run a PR or crush a new distance, we often get unrealistically optimistic at the start of the race.

We think maybe, just maybe, all of our training has suddenly peaked at mythical proportions and we can run faster than we have ever run before.

Another common experience is that we just want to break free of the crowds at the beginning of the race so we are not held back. We just want to run our own race!

One masters runner, Jeremy, told me a story of a 5k race he ran where he purposely wanted to start the race faster to get around some slower runners that were blocking his way. He did get ahead of the slower runners, but he ended up paying the price later.

I can't help but think that those slower runners Jeremy was trying to avoid actually could have been beneficial. Perhaps if he had used them to pace his first mile slower, that final mile would have been faster and less painful, and the following section explains why.

The Positives of the Negative Split Strategy

If you start running at your goal pace from the gun, you have not given your body enough time to warm up and settle into the race. The nervous energy, adrenaline, and other feel-good hormones haven't had a chance to fully circulate and be beneficial to your effort. You might start breathing more rapidly than you would have had you eased into the pace. Mentally, you may feel more frantic and panicked than you would if you had started a little less aggressively, and mental stress is just as impactful as physical stress, which just further compounds the effort as you run.

So for the first quarter of the race, it's far better to be much slower than goal pace to ensure that your muscles and your brain are ready to peak later in the race when things get much harder.

Additionally, your body is not at its best until about the middle of the race, so pushing hard at the beginning will only make the second half more difficult. Because your body is primed for performance mid race IF you start slower, a negative split is actually easier to achieve than you might think.

I will add that even splits as opposed to negative splits can also be a very effective strategy. The concept of even splits is nearly the same as negative splits because the effort to stay even rises as the race goes on. But I would argue that staying even the entire race is more challenging and takes greater skill because there is so little room for error. By starting off slower than goal pace, you have more room to adjust as the race unfolds.

Now if it were easy to execute a negative split just because I told you to do it, I could end this section right here. But simple and easy aren't the same thing, so let's break down how you can actually achieve it.

How to Practice a Negative Split in Training

The first step is practice. Just like everything running, the more you practice, the better you will be when it counts.

This does not mean that you should try to finish every single run faster than you started, but you can try practicing first on your easy runs. Easy runs should ALWAYS start very slow. Not just easy, but very slow. You are simply jogging for the first 10 to 15 minutes at a very leisurely pace. This allows blood to start flowing, bringing oxygen to your muscles, and your heart to gradually start beating faster instead of suddenly.

As you start to get into the groove of your easy run, you can allow your pace to speed up, but your final mile should still be well in your easy zone. If you don't know what easy means for you, I recommend you try closing your mouth. If you can run several minutes breathing only out of your nose, then you are going easy.

Finish Fast in Workouts

The next place to practice negative splitting is in your speed workouts. Even if you are not training for a specific race, making sure your last rep is the fast rep is a great idea. The trick to executing this is not by focusing on how fast the last lap needs to be but by making sure the first lap is much slower.

Now, I know that runners absolutely HATE this advice. When I assign them to go to the track, they want to make the most of it and crush the workout start to finish. But I promise, the most reliable way to make your final rep better than the first is to consciously run the first few just a little slower than you think you should. And if by the end of the workout, you have a ton of juice left, by all means, give it what you've got at the end. Just don't do it at the beginning.

You can also practice running faster on tired legs by adding some speed at the end of some of your long runs. While the main goal of a long run is to boost your aerobic capacity, finishing fast is also a skill that needs to be polished. For example, if you have a 12 mile long run, try running the first 8 miles nice and easy and goal half marathon pace for the next 3 miles, and then slow down to a jog for the final mile as a cool-down.

Be Realistic With Your Goal Time

With workouts and easy runs going well, you should start to be able to come up with a finish time estimate that is reasonable for your next race. We never know what will happen on race day, of course, but aiming for a slightly more conservative finish time than your training indicates can help you pull off the negative split strategy, and perhaps cross the finish line faster than expected.

I believe it's fear of the unknown, doubt, and lack of confidence that hurts our race performances the most. And that's natural! If we don't have a ton of experience racing, we don't know what will happen, so many of us simply say, "I'm going to do my best!" and race without a plan, without a strategy, and without confidence that a strategic plan could actually help us.

Jeremy used to race like that, but now, detailed planning is key. He even programs his watch with heart rate zones and mile splits to ensure he stays right where he wants to be.

I don't think every runner needs to go into quite as much detail as Jeremy does, but if you have gone out too fast in a race in the past, I would certainly recommend that you do sit down and make a solid plan to increase the effort as you go, choosing paces based on what you have done in your workouts.

Use Negative Effort Instead of Pace for Hilly Courses

The one time that negative splits won't work is during a particularly hilly race or one that starts off downhill and ends uphill. You will simply run faster on a downhill with less effort. But that doesn't mean you should completely forget about the negative split strategy. You'll still want to start off at a lower effort and gradually increase as you go; you'll just need to use your effort as a guide instead of your pace.

Ultimately, it's up to you. Would you rather the race start off fast and strong only to be forced to slow long before the finish? Or would you prefer to control your effort from the start and meter out your energy strategically so that you can power across the line with pride?

Negative splitting takes confidence and control, and it can only be achieved by trusting your fitness level and knowing that you can more than make up the few seconds that you lost at the beginning. By making the beginning of the race easier, you are truly making the end of the race easier as well, which could be the key to running the best race of your life.

Should You Use Pace Groups?

I have been a pace leader many times for my local half marathon and helped several runners reach their goal of a sub-two-hour half. This is one of the most rewarding ways to run a race for me, and many runners credit a good pace group for helping them achieve their race goals.

But if you lean too heavily on a group that isn't right for you, it can ruin your race. So how can you decide if a pace group will help or hurt you?

What Is a Pace Group?

Before I discuss the pros and cons, let's talk about exactly what pace groups are. Basically, a pace group is a group of people who are either paid or volunteer to run a race at a certain pace or in a specific finish time. Bigger races will often have them, usually at popular Boston qualifying times or in 15-minute increments or so.

You should be able to find out on the race website if pace groups are being used, and they might even have some of the members of the pace team available to talk to at the expo the day before the race.

In the elite field, hired pacers, called rabbits, run a specific pace so that the athletes following them do not have to concern themselves with strategy or jostling for the lead and can simply hang on, draft, and run.

Some marathons specifically do not allow pacers, such as the Boston Marathon, believing that the sport is more pure when all racers have to simply race. The downside of that is that races without pacers tend to be much slower, as the athletes will more often employ a "wait and kick" strategy, purposely starting off much slower than necessary to avoid the burden of leading too early.

The Chicago Marathon, on the other hand, used rabbits for 26 years before eliminating them in 2015. But by 2018, they were back, because race officials concluded that paced races were simply faster and more exciting.

So if pacers make elites run faster, could using a pace group help you with your goal, too? Yes, if you follow a few tips.

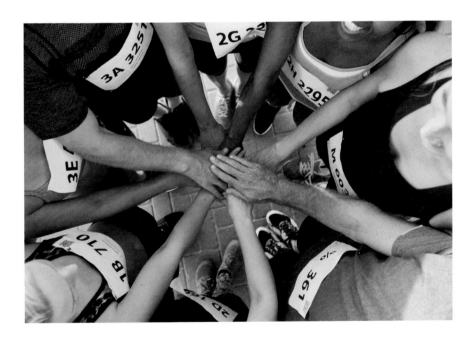

Talk to The Group Leader Before the Race

The single biggest piece of advice I can give you is to find the pace group leader before the race and ask about his or her plan. Here are a few important questions:

- Are you planning to run even splits, despite the terrain, and simply be a visual time clock?
- Will you run by effort, meaning slower on the uphills and faster on the downhills?
- Do you plan to negative split, or run the second half faster than the first?

Make sure that the leader's answers match up with your plan for the race. If not, keep the group's position in view, but run your own race.

You might also ask the leader what their PR is. Is the leader much stronger than the pace he is leading? Or will he be struggling just as much as you?

You want a leader that is much stronger than the pace, but keep in mind that if she miscalculates, she is strong enough to speed up at the end to make the time while you might not be able to.

Pros and Cons for Pace Groups

In one of my full marathons, I ran next to a pacer for the half that was going on simultaneously and asked what his plan was since his splits seemed a little fast by my watch. He actually said that he was planning to put "time in the bank" on the flat course, meaning that he was starting out too fast on purpose! That's the type of pacer you want to avoid, with the possible exception of a course that starts downhill and finishes up on flat.

But once you are satisfied that you have a good pacer, running with a pace group can be very beneficial. You can quiet your brain and just hang on with the group. If it's windy, you can tuck behind and draft. The energy of the group can help minimize the effort you feel, so running at pace feels easier. You can ask the pace leader what to expect, assuming he or she has run the course before, and you can avoid going out too fast by simply sticking with the group.

On the other hand, if you choose to follow a pace group that's a little too ambitious for your fitness level, you could be setting yourself up for a very tough day. If you are in between pace groups, you might not be able to take advantage of them, but it's far better to run your own race than to be overly optimistic and be forced to slow down because you started out in a much faster group than your ability.

In general, pace groups can be enormously helpful, but don't 100 percent rely on them. Make sure you still double check your watch to be sure that you are on target.

I speak from experience on that one. When trying to break three hours in the marathon, I thought I was doing awesome staying with the perfectly paced group. I was so trusting after seeing the even splits each mile that I gave up even looking at my watch. We crossed the half marathon mark in exactly 1:30, and I settled in and tucked behind the pace leader in the wind, giving him my absolute faith and trust that he would bring me home under the line as promised.

When the group pulled away during the final 5k, I thought for sure I was getting slower. I was so sure of it that I didn't look at my watch because I figured I was running as fast as I possibly could, so what did time matter at that point?

Well, that attitude cost me my goal time. I was actually not slowing down that much. The group was speeding up. I missed the sub three by 30 seconds, while my so-called perfect pacer had crossed the line two precious minutes under schedule.

How I Like to Pace

As a pacer myself, I tell everyone around me my plan at the start so they can choose to go with me or not. I prefer to pace the way I coach my athletes to race, letting the terrain set the pace, not just the watch.

If it's a perfectly even, flat course, I would run even splits. On hills, I'll keep the effort the same as flat, which means the pace has to slow on the ups and has to speed up on the downs. Of course, that involves performing math, which is not always easy to do when you are running, but I truly think it's a lot more helpful to pace it like you would race it.

But not every pacer shares my philosophy, and that's okay too. Some pacers believe they should be a visual representation of the clock, much like that world record line you see moving ahead of the swimmers in the Olympics. Just be sure that you know which school of pacing your pacer is following before you follow her.

And hopefully, by using pace groups wisely, you can let the group guide you to your next PR.

How to Ruin Your Running Progress With Too Much Racing

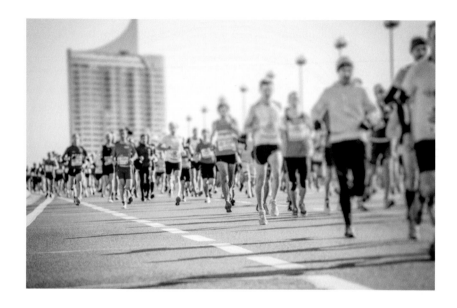

Can you ruin your running progress with too much racing? In a word, yes.

But it doesn't have to be that way. With smart planning (yes, you need a plan!), you can add races to your schedule throughout the year that enhance your fitness level and your ability to race well when it counts the most.

Now you might be wondering why I chose to talk about the topic of over-racing just as some races are finally coming back after the pandemic. But that's EXACTLY why I think this is the perfect time to discuss it.

Races are coming back, and we runners are so thankful and excited to get back to the sport that it's tempting to sign up for any and every race you can.

I'm the last person that is going to tell you that you shouldn't go race, be social, test your fitness level, and hang out with your tribe of runners. If it's bringing you joy, it's probably good for you. We all could use a big dose of joy right now. But if that's how you spend every weekend, and you are wondering why your race times haven't improved in a while, or if they are getting worse, over-racing might have something to do with it.

Before I get into that, let's talk first about the benefits of racing shorter distances in the buildup to a big goal race.

Why Racing Is Awesome

Running hard is HARD, and when you race, that hard effort can feel just a little bit easier. In fact, science has shown that running with others reduces your perception of effort, so you can run faster with others than you can alone.

This is especially true if you do a majority of your hard running by yourself. It's so much better to have competitors along with you to help nudge you to better performances and distract you from the daunting task of running hard for 5k. If you typically have trouble pushing yourself beyond your comfort zone on your own, racing can be some helpful peer pressure.

Racing Tests Your Fitness

Racing is also a great way to measure your progress and your fitness level. One of the hardest things, mentally, about long blocks of training without racing is that it's often difficult to notice if you are improving or not.

I mean, how can you tell if your 10×800 meters this week are on par with or better than your 2x3 mile tempo run last week?

But when you race the same distance over and over, you have a much clearer answer of where your fitness level is during each race. And if those times keep getting faster, it's a major confidence boost that you are doing something right.

Racing Makes You Better at Racing

Another great part about racing in the buildup of training for a more important goal race is that you gain experience racing. Racing is definitely a skill, so incorporating some tune-up races or dress rehearsal races is highly recommended at least once or twice before the real goal race.

If you are training for a long race like the marathon, scheduling a half marathon tune-up race between three and five weeks before your marathon is a great idea to make sure that your race plans for fueling and hydration are actually going to work the way you hope they do.

Racing Is Fun

For many runners, the best part of racing is sharing the love of running with people that love running just as much. Your non-running friends and family just don't get what's so amazing about running, and race events allow you to celebrate your full-on runner-geekiness! These are your people!

It's also a thrill to test your fitness with others and maybe get a medal or an age-group award. At bigger races, you might get to travel to different cities or countries, snag some cool race swag, and hang out with a frosty cold one at the finish line.

The social part of the race environment is a big motivating part of training for many runners. It's what gets you out the door at 5 a.m. when you'd rather stay in bed.

But like most things super fun, racing has a price.

The Downsides of Racing Too Much

Races are harder than regular workouts. The adrenaline is pumping, and the crowd is pushing you to new limits. If you are trying your hardest (which most people are), you are pushing yourself up to and potentially crossing an exertion line that is not sustainable week in and week out.

Extra Recovery Time

Even if you say, "I'm just going to do this race as a tempo run," how many times do you really stick to that plan? If you have any competitive bones in your body, you'll forget what you told yourself and run as hard as you can when the bib is on and the competition is there.

So that means you'll need extra time to recover from that extra effort. The extra recovery time will mean that you can't get back to the training that is specific to your main goal race as quickly, if at all.

Not Specific to Your Goal

If your big goal is a fall marathon, and you spend three out of four weekends over the summer racing other distances, you might get better at those distances, but it will put a major dent in your marathon training. That's because you are sacrificing your marathon-specific work when you are busy racing and recovering.

Are you willing to give up your long run so you can race a 5k? Or are you just going to race the 5k Saturday and plan to run your long run Sunday and hope for the best?

This becomes a slippery slope pretty quickly. If you don't take the extra time to recover from the race, those marathon-specific workouts suffer because you are not ready to run them at your full rested potential. So not only are you not recovering well, but you are also not training well.

Plateauing and the Mental Toll

If you race enough, pay attention to the faces around you. Often, you'll see the same runners over and over again, lining up behind the same pace groups every weekend. They are chasing the same goal time week in and week out and not improving.

Can you imagine what is going on inside of the heads of those runners? What kind of toll would it take on your psyche to keep going after the same goal week after week or month after month and not achieve it?

It's just plain physics that you are not going to be able to improve your race times week after week, so how do you deal with the disappointment of the inevitable bad races over and over again? Racing always involves some risk to the ego, so you better have an ego made of Teflon if you love to race a lot.

Race With a Plan

The key is to find a balance with fun racing and disciplined tune ups or dress rehearsals and dedicate a solid chunk of time to building fitness without racing and the constant pressure to test that fitness all the time.

You can't build fitness if you are always testing it!

Best of Both Worlds

Now if you are agreeing with everything that I've said here, but you still can't bear to be away from the fun and social scene of the race environment, there is another way to get your fill of good running vibes without risking your long term running goals, and that's by volunteering.

I've always had WAY more fun working at a water station and cheering on runners than I ever did racing for myself. If you love racing, why not try subbing one of those races in for a volunteer position? I promise you will love it, and it might just be a better thing for your training and your soul.

Trail Running Tips for Beginners

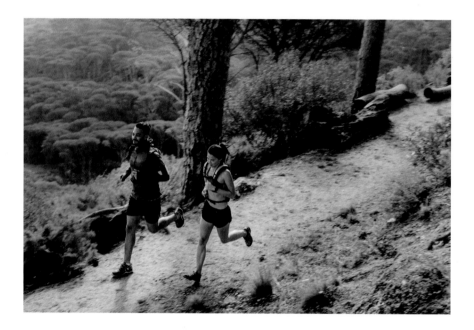

When the weather is hot and the thought of melting into the molten asphalt on a run sounds less than appealing, nothing is better than taking cover in the cool shade of the woods.

Besides being cooler than the hot roads, many people think trail running is cooler in general than dodging BMWs and pausing your Garmin at every stoplight. But if you've never tried it before, trail running can be a little intimidating, so this section is all about tips to get you started.

When I first got into it, my biggest fear wasn't the terrain or the potential for runner-eating animals. I was afraid of getting lost.

So what I did was get on my local running shop's events page and found a regular trail running group that met in the evenings once a week. I showed up at the trail head with a handful of strangers and followed them into the woods for an hour. (I promise, it's not as scary as it sounds.) It was really hard, and I was the one everyone had to wait for at the intersections, but I had a blast and soon became a regular. Because of that group, I made friends, found community, and learned the local trail system so that I could feel comfortable hitting the trails on my own or with groups of my new friends.

Trail-Specific Shoes

The first thing you'll want to have when you hit the trails is a decent pair of trail running shoes. Trail shoes are sturdier, have better rock protection, and provide more traction in mud or on rocks. If your trail is not particularly technical (that is, full of rocks and roots), you can probably get away with using your road shoes for a little while, but if and when you decide that you love trail running, you'll want to invest in a pair that you can feel confident in on any surface.

Be Prepared for Some Falls

But even with the very best trail shoes on the market, be prepared that you will fall at some point. Everyone falls trail running. It's just a fact. And most of the time, you are just fine and can brush it off. I often wear a pair of fingerless gloves when on the trails, even in warm weather, because I'm a serious trail klutz, and they have saved the pads of my hands from scrapes. But most people don't do this and somehow manage to have perfectly uninjured palms.

Obviously, the reason that you might fall is due to the uneven terrain, but most of the time the real culprit is that you've zoned out for a moment and missed that gnarly root snaking across the path. That is another fact about trail running: You have to be in the moment, paying attention at all times. You want to keep your focus about ten feet in front of you so that you can hop, skip, or jump over whatever obstacle comes your way.

Now, I am the type of runner that loves zoning out. I love running the same road over and over again because I'm lost in my mind or listening to a podcast or music.

But trail running teaches you to let your worries and stress go for a while and be literally and truly focused only on what is in front of you at the moment. And that can be a good lesson for the rest of your life as well.

Effort and Time Instead of Pace and Distance

This brings me to another difference between trail and road: Your paces will be much slower. And for some runners, that's tough to accept. Of course it makes sense that if you are climbing up and down a mountain that you will be slower than you would be if running on a track, but it can be hard to look at your watch after a two hour long trail run only to find you ran half as far as you guessed you did. And yet you are twice as sore.

So you need to go by effort instead of pace and time instead of distance. I am always preaching about how effort is king to my athletes, and nowhere is that more true than in the woods. You can run a 16-minute mile that feels every bit as hard as an 8-minute mile on flat, and to your body, it is pretty much the same thing. So it can be helpful to measure your run by time and elevation change instead of pace and distance if you are the measuring type (and c'mon, we all are, right?).

A lot of runners prefer the trails because they feel the softer dirt surface is easier on their bodies than the roads. From an injury point of view, trail runners are no less likely to get hurt than roadies, so it's not a magic bullet, but it can be nice to vary up the surfaces of your runs to help avoid overuse injuries.

But the key thing to remember is that, on trails, you are not simply moving forward. You are dodging rocks and roots and leaping over small streams, so different ancillary muscles are going to be engaged. And that's why you might feel sore after your first trail run, even if you are a strong road runner. You'll find muscles you didn't know existed before.

To help prevent that, strength training to the rescue. Strength training should be standard fare for every type of runner, but trail runners want to be sure that they are getting lateral or side to side strength training as well as plyometrics for power.

Leave No Trace

Once you are on the trail, you want to be sure that you are practicing proper trail etiquette. First and foremost, don't litter. I hope you are not doing that on the roads, either, but it's especially important in the woods. Put those used gel wrappers back in your pockets and toss them out at home. If you see someone else's trash, be kind and pick it up!

Share the Trail

When approaching another runner on a single track, make room so you can both pass. Stay to the right, just like you would when driving (at least in places that drive on the right!). If runners are heading your direction and the trail is too narrow to share, the runner(s) on the uphill side of the trail should step off and let those on the downhill side pass before continuing.

Avoid startling others, and enable them to make room for you by shouting a quick "on your left" as you pass them from behind. If you are on a trail shared by mountain bikes or horses, yield to them, because you can stop more easily.

Some people's greatest fear about trail running is encountering animals. First of all, most animals don't want anything to do with you, and animal attacks on trail runners are extremely rare. The best way to avoid encounters is to be loud and bright. Making noise, shuffling leaves, singing and talking, or even running with a bell or a whistle all make the animals want to avoid you. (The same is true for people, too, but I digress.) Not wearing headphones is also a great idea so that you are more aware of your surroundings.

But if you are still unsure, learn about the potential animal threats in your area and the best way to deal with each species so that you are armed with knowledge before you run.

Trail running can be a great way to add some variety to your running, or it might completely take over your running all together. It can seem intimidating at first, but there is a very good reason that it's becoming more and more popular. Going for a run, alone or with friends, in places that are only accessible by foot is a beautifully human experience that you can enjoy all year round.

Chapter Ten

Planted Runner Recipes

While I generally rely on my much-loved cookbooks to create delicious plant-based meals, there are some recipes that I just had to come up with myself! Commercial running products are certainly convenient, but they can also be expensive and wasteful to rely on all the time. Here I share some of my favorite running recipes made famous on my blog, theplantedrunner.com.

Electrolyte Replacement Hydration

If you are running or racing in the heat for longer than an hour, replacing the electrolytes you've lost in your sweat is essential. Ideally, you should drink water and replace the electrolytes with real food at the end of your run. But sometimes, you want to hydrate and replenish lost electrolytes in one drink.

NUUN is a convenient commercial product that achieves this, and I have my own copy-cat version.

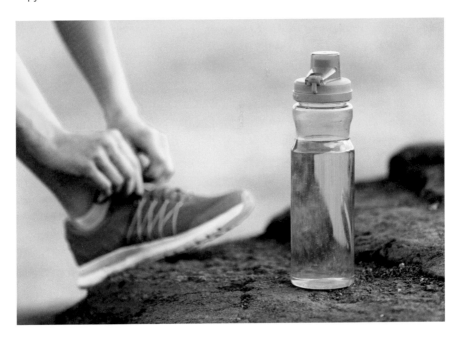

DIY NUUN Electrolyte Replacement

Makes one 16 ounce serving

Ingredients
1/4 teaspoon baking soda (307mg sodium)
1/16 teaspoon Morton's Lite Salt (87.5mg potassium and 72.5mg sodium)
1/16 teaspoon epsom salt (30mg magnesium)
Optional flavor such as juice, tea, stevia, or water enhancer

Measure directly into 16 ounces of cold still or sparkling water or other beverage.
Each serving contains 372.5 mg sodium 87.5 mg potassium 30 mg magnesium

Race Fuel

There are many different products on the market designed to fuel your running and your racing. Store-bought options are convenient, but they can be expensive. I've come up with several recipes that you can make at home for much less!

DIY Generation UCAN

This recipe fueled my sub-three-hour marathon in Phoenix with no tummy issues!

First a little background on UCAN. Generation UCAN is a modified cornstarch and flavoring mix that you add to water. It costs around $2 per serving, and you can make an alternative for pennies!

It was developed initially to treat people with a rare condition called glycogen storage disease (GDS). People with this life-threatening condition cannot properly store glycogen and their blood glucose levels fall to dangerous levels while they sleep.

In 1984, it was discovered that ingesting plain, uncooked cornstarch before bed kept patients' glucose levels in the desired range and dramatically improved their lives, many of them children. The only problem with uncooked cornstarch therapy? After about 4.5 hours, glucose levels start to fall, and a second dose is required. Parents still had to wake up their children in the middle of the night to feed them.

So the scientists came up with a modified form of cornstarch that kept glucose levels stable for 8 to 10 hours, and patients could finally sleep through the night. Then someone had the bright idea to apply the technology to another group of people who struggle with maintaining steady glycogen levels: endurance athletes.

And UCAN was born. UCAN claims that because starch empties the stomach quickly and is slowly but completely absorbed into the bloodstream that it is very gentle on the stomach.

But unless you need 8 to 10 hours to run a marathon without refueling, my regular cornstarch recipe will work great!

How does my homemade UCAN alternative version compare to lemon UCAN? A single-serving packet of lemon UCAN (not the scoop) contains 28 grams of carbohydrate, 110 calories, 230mg sodium, and 140mg potassium.

My version is 30 grams of carbohydrate, 136 calories, 219mg sodium, and 87mg potassium plus a small amount of magnesium and calcium. I'm not going to pretend it's as delicious as a fresh-squeezed lemonade (neither is UCAN), but it is not bad at all, just has a slight chalkiness texture.

DIY Generation UCAN

Makes two 8-ounce servings

Ingredients
8 2/3 tbsp (70g) cornstarch or tapioca flour
1 packet True Lemon drink enhancer
1/8 tsp salt
1/8 tsp Morton's Lite Salt
16 oz water

Mix all ingredients together and pour into two 8-ounce fuel bottles. Cornstarch will settle to the bottom, so be sure to give it a shake before drinking.

Each serving contains 120 calories, 30g carbohydrate, 219mg sodium, 87 mg potassium.

Sugar-Free Chocolate Milk Race Fuel

Makes one 4-ounce serving

Ingredients
1/4 cup (40g) cornstarch or tapioca flour
1 teaspoon (2g) cocoa powder
1/16 teaspoon salt
1/16 teaspoon Morton's Lite Salt
10 drops liquid vanilla stevia
4 ounces of water (more if a thinner consistency is desired)

Mix all ingredients together and pour into two 8-ounce fuel bottles. Cornstarch will settle to the bottom, so be sure to give it a shake before drinking.

Each serving contains 153 calories, 38g carbohydrate, 219mg sodium, 87 mg potassium.

Endurance Gels

One of the most common questions I get from plant-based athletes is how can you fuel mid-run with real food? Some athletes happily fuel themselves with packets of maple syrup, handfuls of dried fruit, or squeeze packs of applesauce. I've come up with a few more options!

I do need to warn you, however, that not everyone's stomach can handle digesting real food when they are running hard. Simple sugars and starches without fiber often are gentler on the stomach, which is why I've included some recipes that include pure corn syrup. I encourage you to experiment and see what works best for you.

Brownie Batter Endurance Gel

Makes 2 gels

Ingredients
4 medjool dates with the pits removed, soaked overnight if not already soft
4 ounces of water
1/8 teaspoon salt
2 teaspoon cocoa powder

Blend all ingredients together very well. I prefer to use an immersion blender since that's the easiest to clean, especially for small quantities. Add more liquid as desired to create the consistency that you like. Once the gel is smooth, pour into a gel flask, food-safe silicone travel bottle, or seal in custom FoodSaver bags. Store in freezer until ready to use.

Each gel contains 144 calories, 37g of carbohydrate, 150mg of sodium, 307mg potassium.

Apple Pie Endurance Gel

Makes 2 gels

Ingredients
1 tablespoon frozen apple juice concentrate
3 tablespoons pure corn syrup (Karo is a good brand)
1 tablespoon agave syrup
1/8 teaspoon salt
1/8 teaspoon cinnamon
1/8 teaspoon ground ginger

Mix all ingredients together well and pour into a gel flask, food-safe silicone travel bottle, or seal in custom FoodSaver bags. Store in freezer until ready to use.

Each gel contains 147 calories, 34g of carbohydrate, 173mg of sodium.

Margarita Endurance Gel

Makes 2 gels

Ingredients
2 tablespoons pure corn syrup (not high fructose)
1 tablespoon agave syrup
1/2 teaspoon salt
2 teaspoons lime juice

Mix all ingredients together well and pour into a gel flask, food-safe silicone travel bottle, or seal in custom FoodSaver bags. Store in freezer until ready to use.

Each gel contains 92 calories, 23.5g of carbohydrate, 173mg of sodium.

Post-Run Snacks

The goal with your post-run food is replenishment and recovery. You want to refill your glycogen stores with carbohydrate, restock the electrolytes lost in your sweat, and help your muscles repair with protein. I go into this in more detail in chapter one, but here are a few of my favorites.

Gingerbread Truffles

Makes 12 truffles, 2 per serving

Ingredients
1/2 cup almond meal or ground almonds
1/2 cup cashew meal or ground cashews
1/2 cup natural peanut butter or peanut flour
1 cup pitted medjool dates
1 teaspoon ground ginger
1 teaspoon black strap molasses
1 1/2 teaspoons vanilla extract
1-4 tablespoons water (as needed)
Cocoa or cacao powder for rolling

If you already have almond or cashew meal (Trader Joe's sells them), add all ingredients except the water and cocoa to a food processor and blend until you achieve a cookie-dough consistency, adding water one tablespoon at a time if needed to make dough (if you use peanut flour—I like PB Fit—you will need to add a couple tablespoons or more of water).

If you are starting from whole nuts, grind those first into a fine meal before adding the other ingredients, being careful not to overprocess into nut butter.

Once you have a sticky dough, dust your clean hands and a plate with cocoa powder. Roll the dough into bite-size truffles coated with cocoa.

These keep best in the fridge but should be fine without refrigeration for several hours (if they last that long!).

Each two-truffle serving contains 58 calories, 4.6g fat, 2.8g carbs, 1.6g protein.

Walnut Artichoke Pesto Salad

Makes 4 servings

Ingredients
14 ounces canned or jarred marinated artichoke hearts, undrained
1 cup packed cilantro
3/4 cup walnuts
3 cloves garlic
2 tablespoons lemon juice
3/4 teaspoon sea salt
3/4 teaspoon ground pepper

Throw everything into the food processor and pulse until you have a chunky pesto.

Serve on top of mixed greens with whatever veggies you like. Or, use as a dip for bread or toasted pita.

Each serving contains 163 calories, 13g fat, 9g carbs, 5g protein.

Hot Blackstrap Molasses Cocoa

Many runners, especially plant-based runners, need to find ways to incorporate more iron into their diets. Blackstrap molasses is naturally rich in iron and when paired with fortified plant-based milk, it makes a rich, nutrient-dense cocoa. Perfect after a cold run!

Ingredients
10 ounces almond milk or other fortified plant milk
1 tablespoon blackstrap molasses
1 tablespoon cocoa powder
1 teaspoon vanilla extract
Pinch of salt

Heat almond milk over the stove or in the microwave. Stir in the remaining ingredients until dissolved. Enjoy!

Each serving has 100 calories, 14.7 g carbs, 3.5g fat, 2.2g protein, 648mg potassium, 344mg sodium, 32% RDA Vitamin A, 74% RDA calcium, and 30.4% RDA iron.